THE HUMAN TOUCH IN MODERN MEDICINE

Putting "Care" back at the Centre of Health Care

THE HUMAN TOUCH IN MODERN MEDICINE

Putting "Care" back at the Centre of Health Care

By

Dr. Gourdas Choudhuri

Qurate
qaratebooks.com

The Human Touch in Modern Medicine
Dr Gourdas Choudhuri

Published in 2025

© Published by

Qurate Books Pvt. Ltd.
Goa 403523, India
www.quratebooks.com
Tel: 1800-210-6527, Email: info@quratebooks.com

ISBN: 978-93-58989-30-4

Acknowledgements

There are two persons who touched me and impacted my life most: one was my maternal grandfather, Mr AC Moitra, who brought me up through my difficult childhood, for whom "kindness was not an act, but a reflection of the soul" and showed that "the best portion of a man's life is his little, nameless unremembered acts of kindness and love". The other was my high school teacher, Fr AP Roberts, who encouraged me to question myself at every turn and keep observing the path I was treading, by looking OVER any prism, rather than THROUGH one.

Every since I became a doctor, my patients and their relatives became my best teachers, indicating in their subtle ways, what endeared and touched them, as well as what hurt their feelings. It is not unusual for patients to show their gratitude through cards or cakes if the treatment has gone well; what I valued most however were grateful words and blessings from relatives of a patient I was caring for who had died!

The "science" of medicine requires a doctor to be professional, objective and impersonal so that emotions do not cloud clinical judgement. A saying however goes, "It is a "good" doctor who diagnoses and treats the disease, but it is a "great" doctor who treats the patient who has the disease".

My wife, Arundhati, has been a pillar of support in my human engagements all through my professional life, and put up boldly with the unimaginable pressures and stress that she had to face as a doctor's spouse.

This book would not have been possible without the untiring help and support of Nitika Nagpal, who was once a patient herself, but felt inspired to participate in spreading compassion.

I thank my friends and colleagues Dr. Shiv K Sarin and Dr. Raghuvanshi for their forewords. Ajey Maharaj and Milind helped out at various stages and many others who contributed to this first baby-step towards a big cause.

Gourdas

About the Author

Dr. Gourdas Choudhuri (MD, DM, FACG, FRCP, FAMS, WHO-fellow) is a medical specialist, teacher, researcher, philanthropist and writer.

He graduated from JIPMER, Pondicherry, and trained at the All India institute of Medical Sciences, New Delhi. Through fellowships and friendships he trained and observed patient-doctor relationships from several regions of India, Nagoya University, Japan, Kreiskrankenhaus Völklingen, Germany, University of Sydney, Australia", but retained and nurtured his connect with the innumerable Indian patients he served in India.

During his over 42 years as a medical specialist, Dr. Choudhuri has been professor and head of Gastroenterology at the Sanjay Gandhi Postgraduate Institute of Medical Sciences, Lucknow, President of the National Indian Society of Gastroenterology, and has played a leadership role in developing liver and digestive healthcare in the country.

He strongly believes that awareness on health issues, helps individuals live better and tackle challenges more efficiently and effectively when they arise. His passion led him to create Hope Initiative (www.hope.org.in) in 2004 through which he campaigned to including health as a component of school education. He has written a health column called ***Health Adda*** for 13 years.

He lives in Gurgaon and provides medical services in Gurgaon and Lucknow.

To know more about him visit www.drgchoudhuri.net

Foreword

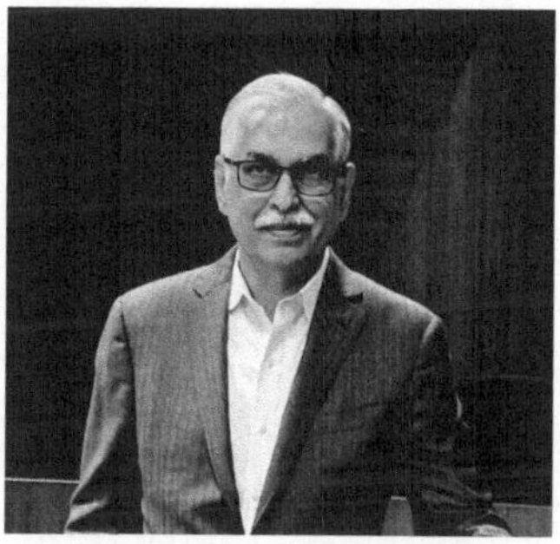

Dr. Gourdas Choudhuri's "**The Human Touch in Modern Medicine**" serves as a vital reminder of the core principles that should guide healthcare: empathy, understanding, and compassion. Amidst the remarkable advances in medical science and technology, this book reinforces the importance of maintaining a focus on caring for people, not just treating diseases.

Articulating the balance between leveraging technological advancements and nurturing personal connections essential for true healing, Dr. Choudhuri emphasizes that, even in an age of medical breakthroughs, the human element remains irreplaceable.

This book offers invaluable lessons for anyone involved in the healthcare industry. Through practical advice and inspiring examples, Dr. Choudhuri illustrates how integrating compassion into daily medical practice can greatly enhance patient care and lead to better health outcomes.

I highly recommend this book to healthcare providers, educators, and policymakers. It serves as a powerful guide for enriching patient interactions and underscores the crucial role of humanity in healthcare. May the insights from this book inspire us all to foster a more empathetic and caring approach in our work.

Dr. Ashutosh Raghuvanshi

MD & CEO, Fortis Healthcare

Foreword

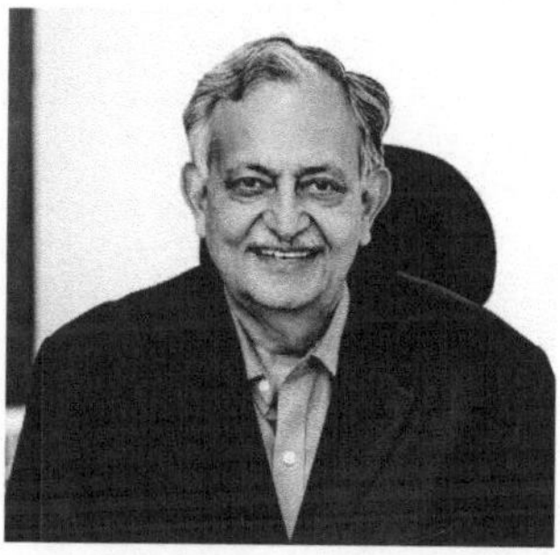

Filled with real life stories, throbbing with emotions, seamless learnings, the book, "**The Human Touch in Modern Medicine**" by Dr. Gourdas is a masterpiece. The narrations in the book, reflect multitudes of learnings of a master clinician and a rare human being. The book makes the reader appreciate, how a great doctor feels and lives his life. Medicine is one of the most difficult profession, as the doctor has to live several lives at the same moment; the patient's, his/her relatives', the society, his professional knowledge and ethics and his inner emotions. The world assesses the doctor on the first four. The book by Dr. Choudhuri, speaks about the fifth, the need for emotional maturation of the doctor, the key to healing, the human touch. The empathy, the compassion, the humane aspects of medicine are indeed the core of healing and medicine. He recounts memorable anecdotes from his experience, laced with reasoning, which reflect what the patients want. The narrated parables succinctly describe the dilemmas which a doctor, a healer faces. No profession other than medicine poses multitudes of ethical challenges everyday; is it right or wrong, should I do it or not! The writings in this priceless treasure gave me several new thoughts and learnings to improve my life and practice of medicine. The book also serves as an eye-opener to the general public, to know how doctor's make decisions, which even if not favorable to the patient or relative, are most often, full of care and empathy.

'The Human Touch in Modern Medicine', is a poignant disposition of humanity at its best, and a real treat to be read by one and all. It enriches yours soul, heals your heart, makes your vision saintly and turns you into a better human being. Possess it and adorn your book-shelf.

Dr. Shiv K Sarin

Director, ILBS and President, National Academy of Medical Sciences

Chairman Medical Council of India (MCI), 2010-2011

Contents

Why should you read this book?

"Wherever the art of medicine is loved, there is also a love of humanity"
Socrates

The 21st century presents a profound paradox in the medical profession: it is simultaneously experiencing an era of unprecedented advancement and a period of significant challenge. We stand at the pinnacle of both medical knowledge and technological innovation, witnessing breakthroughs that were once considered science fiction.

The Explosion of Medical Knowledge and Technology

In the last few decades there has been an explosion of medical knowledge and technology, transforming our ability to diagnose, treat, and prevent disease. Vaccines have eradicated or significantly reduced the prevalence of once-feared illnesses. Antibiotics have revolutionized the treatment of bacterial infections. Rapid and reliable diagnostic tools, such as advanced imaging and genetic testing, allow for earlier and more precise diagnoses. These advancements have collectively contributed to longer and healthier lifespans for countless individuals.

Furthermore, medical innovation has extended far beyond infectious diseases. Organ transplantation has become a life-saving option for patients with failing organs, offering a second chance at life. Minimally invasive surgical techniques have reduced recovery times and patient discomfort. Joint replacements have restored mobility and improved the quality of life for millions. Even in the fight against cancer, significant progress has been made, with new therapies and targeted treatments offering hope and extending survival rates.

Yet alongside these remarkable achievements, a disquieting trend has emerged, threatening the very foundation of the doctor-patient relationship.

The Depersonalization of Patient Care

This remarkable progress has been accompanied by a troubling side effect: the depersonalization of patient care. In the fast-paced environment of modern medicine, patients are often reduced to their diagnoses, test results, or room numbers. The phrase "the gallbladder in room 6" or "the COPD in ward B" exemplifies this dehumanizing trend, where patients are treated as cases rather than individuals with unique experiences, fears, and needs. This erosion of personalized care has contributed to a decline in trust and respect for healthcare professionals.

The Double-Edged Sword of Success: Heightened Expectations and Defensive Medicine

Medical science has, in a sense, become a victim of its own success. The dramatic rescues and miraculous recoveries made possible by modern medicine have created a culture of heightened expectations. Instances of patients being brought back from the brink of death, such as the widely publicized cases of athletes like Christian Eriksen and Damar Hamlin who experienced sudden cardiac arrest on the field, are often perceived as the universal new standard. While these stories are undoubtedly inspiring, they can inadvertently set unrealistic expectations for outcomes in other situations. Consequently, any death, especially from a common condition like heart disease, can be mistakenly interpreted as a failure of the medical profession, regardless of the individual circumstances or the complexity of the case.

These elevated expectations can have counterproductive consequences, fostering a climate of blame and defensiveness. Healthcare workers, fearing recrimination and potential litigation, may become hesitant to take necessary risks or pursue innovative approaches, even when these actions could have benefited some of the patients. This phenomenon, known as defensive medicine, can stifle innovation and ultimately compromise patient care. The fear of negative repercussions can even extend beyond the medical setting, with bystanders potentially avoiding helping accident victims to avoid legal entanglements.

The Shift from Holistic Care to Technical Focus

The focus of healthcare has gradually shifted from holistic patient well-being—including physical, mental, and emotional health—to a more technical and outcome-oriented approach. The emphasis is now on diagnostic accuracy, treatment options, predictable outcomes, and extended lifespans. Some argue that with the advent of sophisticated diagnostic tools and standardized treatment protocols, such as laparoscopic cholecystectomy, the role of interpersonal skills and empathy has diminished. This perspective prioritizes scientific knowledge, technical expertise, and measurable outcomes over the human connection essential to the therapeutic relationship.

The Eroding Doctor-Patient Bond

The traditional doctor-patient bond, once characterized by trust, empathy, and open communication, is weakening. To fully understand this growing disconnect despite the remarkable advancements of modern medicine, we must carefully examine the underlying causes and their far-reaching impact on public perception and expectations from the medical profession.

The Imperative of Humanizing Medicine: Restoring Trust and Compassion

If modern medicine's once-unquestioned authority and public trust are beginning to falter, reintroducing empathy, compassion, and a focus on the "human experience" of illness is crucial for restoring its reputation and effectiveness. In essence, "humanizing" medicine is not just a desirable goal; it is an essential imperative.

This book aims to persuade you, the reader, to reconnect with your own humanity and to prioritize the "human" element in your patient care, seeing the distraught frightened patient who has come with a disease seeking your help, rather than merely applying the appropriate tests and techniques that treat just the disease

It will delve into the profound impact of compassionate understanding and empathy on patient recovery, demonstrating how these qualities can significantly enhance the healing process in ways that knowledge and technology cannot; it is even more crucial for patients who are often facing fear, uncertainty, and emotional distress alongside their physical ailments. A human-centred approach, also restores the vital trust and respect for the profession that are essential for the practice of medicine.

Foundations of Healthcare

The Three Pillars of Healthcare

" Nothing is more important than empathy for another human being's suffering. Not a career. Not wealth. Not intelligence. Certainly not status. We have to feel for one another if we're going to survive with dignity"

Audrey Hepburn

It's regrettable that healthcare in recent times is often perceived as solely reliant on medical knowledge, neglecting the crucial roles of interpersonal skills and empathy, which together constitute a vital three-pillar foundation.

In earlier eras, when medical technology and treatments were less advanced, physicians and healthcare workers (HCWs) not only addressed patients' physical ailments but also prioritized establishing rapport, fostering trust and confidence, practicing meticulous clinical observation, providing supportive care encompassing nutrition and hydration, diligently monitoring patient progress, communicating effectively with patients and their families, offering motivation and emotional support, and bolstering their ability to cope with prolonged illnesses or adverse outcomes.

Empathy, the capacity to comprehend the feelings and deep concerns of patients and their loved ones, served as the essential bond between doctor and family, often forging lifelong connections, hence the traditional concept of the "family doctor."

However, in contemporary practice, the fundamental elements of empathy and strong interpersonal relationships are frequently absent from medical curricula and training in many nations, including India. Furthermore, opportunities to learn these crucial humanistic skills by observing experienced teachers are scarce, as many educators themselves have advanced primarily through academic and scientific achievements, sometimes inadvertently serving as inadequate models of compassionate care.

Societal attitudes and behaviour have also undergone significant change. Many contemporary doctors feel that the substantial investment of time, effort, and financial resources (often provided by parents) that have gone into their training should yield commensurate "return on investment." Consequently, the traditionally self-sacrificing "missionary" approach to medicine may appear outdated in the current climate. The escalating costs of living expenses, marriage, homeownership, raising of children, and meeting modern family expectations have become challenging. Moreover, present society seems to have reoriented its values, often prioritizing wealth and material success, as yard sticks of success. Altruistic individuals who have remained poor are sometimes overlooked, disregarded, or even labelled as failures.

Therefore, it is not surprising that an academically successful student, graduating with high grades and honours, may not prioritize empathy, compassion and care.

The need would be to integrate these values in the practice of medicine at all levels, including hi-tech modern medicine.

Empathy: The Distinguishing Badge of Healthcare

What you want to ignite in others must first burn inside yourself.

-Charlotte Brontë

There's no question that a career as a physician or healthcare worker (nurse, physiotherapist, etc.) can be profoundly rewarding. This fulfilment stems from the deep satisfaction of helping those in dire need, suffering, or facing the prospect of death.

Studies have demonstrated that the greatest sense of gratification comes from aiding others in need, surpassing even the pursuit of wealth.

Empathy has long been recognized as a cornerstone of healthcare. These are not fleeting, thrilling sensations like winning a lottery or bungee jumping, where risk and adventure provide entertainment, triggering adrenaline and dopamine surges.

The acts of helping and giving offer a different kind of reward: a sense of satisfaction, meaning, and purpose. Experts on happiness emphasize that these deeper feelings are more strongly correlated with lasting happiness than the temporary surges of dopamine and adrenaline associated with games and thrills.

What is EMPATHY?

Empathy means the ability to recognize and understand what the patient is feeling. It is different from SYMPATHY, which means "feeling sorry or pity" for a person who is suffering.

Empathy is what generates trust and forms the bridge between a distressed patient, who has come seeking help, and me as a doctor, who needs to begin with the reassurance that "I understand" your problem and your feelings.

Distinguished psychologists Daniel Goleman and Paul Ekman have identified three distinct components of empathy: Cognitive, Emotional, and Compassionate.

1. **Cognitive empathy involves being aware of another person's or patient's emotional state. A medical consultation should not be a purely clinical exchange of information and advice, devoid of emotional awareness. It's crucial to discern whether the patient—or a family member, such as a parent—is experiencing anxiety, fear, anger, suspicion, or despair.**
2. **Emotional empathy entails engaging with and sharing those emotions. If a patient expresses fear of having cancer, connecting with them on that emotional level is essential for determining the appropriate tests to alleviate their concerns. Simply writing a prescription is insufficient.**
3. **Compassionate empathy involves taking action to support the patient. For example, if a patient is expressing anger due to perceived delays in addressing their medical issue, directly intervening by ensuring urgent administration of an injection or IV drip can make a significant positive difference.**

Arguing with an agitated patient by demanding patience or suggesting they seek another doctor is guaranteed to damage the patient-doctor relationship and be perceived as uncaring.

Compassionate care should be the essence of healthcare—care delivered not merely with politeness and professionalism, but with genuine empathy and compassion, where your words, facial expressions, and actions convey a sincere interest in the patient's well-being.

Many colleagues and trainees struggle to grasp the importance of professional service combined with compassionate care.

The following example illustrates this point: When requesting water from a flight attendant, they promptly provide it with a professional demeanour and a smile. However, consider a patient with advanced cancer who is experiencing pain, depression, and low morale, and needs their PICC line changed or cleaned. While technical proficiency is essential, simply performing the procedure efficiently is not enough. Understanding how a comforting smile and reassuring presence can instill trust, enhance acceptance, and satisfaction in such a vulnerable patient is the mark of a truly empathetic and compassionate healthcare provider.

Empathy seems to come naturally to some individuals. Research explores the potential genetic basis of empathy, noting its tendency to run in families, with empathetic healthcare workers often having empathetic parents and children.

However, current selection criteria for aspiring healthcare workers and doctors prioritize knowledge and academic merit, neglecting inherent traits like "nature" and "attitude." This raises a crucial question: Can those lacking inherent empathy be taught, trained, or sensitized to develop it?

Fortunately, research indicates that empathy can be learned and cultivated. This involves teaching, discussion, demonstration, and practice. Exposing healthcare professionals to stories, movies, or other media that evoke empathy can also be beneficial.

In today's climate of strained patient-doctor relationships, re-emphasizing empathy is crucial. It is the key differentiator between simply "providing care" and truly "caring."

Emotional Quotient In Healthcare: A Critical Component Of Effective Patient Care

It was not the truth they wanted but an illusion they could bear to live with.

-Anaïs Nin

Emotional Quotient (EQ), or Emotional Intelligence (EI), is the capacity to recognize, understand, and manage one's own emotions and those of others. In the demanding field of healthcare, where professionals frequently encounter stressful situations and emotionally charged interactions, a high EQ is essential. It not only elevates the quality of patient care but also contributes to the well-being of healthcare professionals themselves.

EQ significantly impacts the patient-provider relationship. Professionals with high EQ are better at empathizing with patients, understanding their concerns, and responding supportively and therapeutically. This empathetic approach cultivates trust and enhances communication, leading to more accurate diagnoses and effective treatment plans.

For instance, a provider with high EQ can detect a patient's anxiety or fear, even if unspoken. By addressing these emotions, the provider can alleviate distress, fostering comfort and treatment adherence. This emotional awareness can distinguish between a patient who feels heard and cared for and one who feels overlooked and misunderstood.

Furthermore, high EQ enables healthcare professionals to navigate difficult conversations, such as discussing terminal diagnoses or end-of-life care. In these sensitive situations, conveying empathy, providing support, and managing one's own emotional responses are crucial for delivering compassionate care.

Healthcare is a demanding profession, often involving long hours, high-stress environments, and exposure to suffering and death. These factors can contribute to burnout, characterized by emotional exhaustion, depersonalization, and a diminished sense of personal accomplishment. However, professionals with high EQ are better equipped to handle these emotional demands.

High EQ helps professionals recognize and regulate their own emotions, preventing the accumulation of stress and frustration that can lead to burnout. It also strengthens their ability to build supportive relationships with colleagues, crucial in team-based healthcare settings. By promoting a positive work environment and maintaining their own emotional well-being, professionals with high EQ are more resilient and better positioned to deliver high-quality care.

Recognizing the importance of EQ in healthcare, many medical schools and institutions are incorporating emotional intelligence training into their curricula. This training often includes self-awareness exercises, communication skills workshops, and stress management techniques.

Self-awareness is fundamental to EQ. Healthcare professionals must recognize their own emotional states and understand how these emotions can influence their behavior and interactions with patients. Techniques like mindfulness, reflection, and journaling can aid in developing this essential self-awareness.

As a doctor, you need to be aware and conscious of your own emotional state, so that you can better 'sense' the emotional state of your patient.

Beyond self-awareness, effective communication is crucial for high EQ. Healthcare providers must cultivate active listening skills, respond with empathy, and communicate clearly and compassionately, even during difficult interactions. Training often incorporates role-playing and simulations to provide a safe space for practicing these skills.

Stress management is another vital element of EQ. Healthcare professionals need to develop coping strategies to manage the emotional demands of their work. These strategies can include mindfulness practices, physical exercise, or participation in peer support groups. Effective stress management allows providers to maintain emotional equilibrium and consistently deliver high-quality care.

***

As the healthcare landscape evolves, particularly with increasing technology and telemedicine, EQ's importance will only amplify. While technology enhances efficiency and accessibility, it can also hinder emotional connection and communication. Providers must adapt their EQ skills to these new interaction modes, ensuring empathetic and compassionate care remains central, even in digital environments.

Furthermore, with the growing emphasis on patient-centred care, demand for high-EQ providers will continue to rise. Today's patients expect not only clinical expertise but also emotional support and understanding. Those who can deliver both will be best equipped to meet patient needs and excel in their careers.

Patients come to you not just for your medical expertise, but also for emotional support, even if they don't express it outright. Its best to start developing a healthy EQ.

Emotional Quotient (EQ) is crucial for effective healthcare, enhancing patient care, mitigating provider burnout, and fostering a more compassionate and supportive environment. As healthcare evolves, EQ's importance will only increase, making it an essential skill for all healthcare providers. By developing and honing their emotional intelligence, healthcare professionals become not only skilled clinicians but also compassionate caregivers who truly connect with their patients.

Communication and Social Skills of Doctors

People start to heal the moment they feel heard

-Cheryl Richardson

My non-medical friends are often surprised to learn that "Communication and Social Skills," fundamental to the patient-doctor relationship, are absent from the Indian medical curriculum.

While the rigorous training required to become a doctor is undeniable, attracting some of the most intelligent and persevering individuals, it's equally undeniable that a lack of formal training in communication and social skills contributes to poor patient-doctor relationships and growing public dissatisfaction with the medical profession.

Most professions involving human interaction, such as management, sales, and marketing, recognize communication's vital role and provide training, evaluation, and assessment in these skills. Doctors, however, spend years acquiring knowledge and honing technical skills like surgery but are then expected to interact with patients without any formal training in essential areas like greeting patients, delivering bad news, responding to anxious relatives, or managing difficult situations following a patient's death.

Doctors typically learn these skills through observing their seniors, perpetuating a cycle of often inadequate training. This glaring void in Indian medical education is further compounded by the fact that even highly knowledgeable teachers often lack effective social skills, empathy, and kindness, inadvertently becoming poor role models for trainees.

Too often, trainees are praised for accurate diagnoses and given high grades as reward for their knowledge, while their interactions with patients are overlooked. Patients are treated as "clinical cases" rather than individuals in need of care. Trainees may precisely recite diagnoses but struggle to recall how the patient felt or what they said beyond their symptoms. The clinical examination may be flawless, but the human connection is often absent, representing a significant failure.

Our assessment system focuses heavily on factual knowledge—diseases, symptoms, treatments, and procedures—while the application of this knowledge in a human context is largely ignored. "Wisdom," in this sense, feels unattainable for many. Brilliant students may excel in exams but struggle to connect with patients, being knowledgeable about the "science" but not the person before them.

Changing this in India is challenging. Many in leadership positions, having risen through a system that often dismisses "soft skills," perpetuate the status quo. In contrast, the West has recognized a need for change. The UK's MRCP exams now include communication and social skills, and the US system assesses how doctors handle difficult patient interactions.

In India, training doctors in communication and social skills is not just important—it's urgent. The doctor-patient relationship, once built on trust and empathy, is rapidly deteriorating. Without change, we risk losing the very essence of medicine.

True wisdom goes beyond mastering medical knowledge; it's about personally understanding and connecting with the person in front of you.

Facilitating Graceful Death

I cannot guarantee you sunshine, but I can promise to stand beside you, no matter how hard it rains..

-Matthew Spenser

Rapid advancements in medical science and technology have had a dual impact on both patients and doctors. These advances have undeniably enabled longer, healthier lives, improving disease prevention and treatment. However, they also present a darker side: sometimes prolonging life and suffering in terminally ill patients, often at immense emotional, physical, and financial costs.

Doctors frequently face a conflict between the imperative to save every life possible and the difficulty in accepting that some patients cannot recover to a meaningful quality of life.

There is the understandable emotional drive to "never give up," and persist until the very end. Yet, experience and prognostic indicators often suggest that simply prolonging suffering—extending life by mere hours or days through life support—is not a desirable outcome.

At this juncture, discussing "comfort care" with the patient's family, allowing for a peaceful and dignified passing, particularly if aligned with the patient's wishes, becomes a crucial consideration.

Suggesting comfort care for a patient beyond recovery can be one of the most compassionate decisions you can make as a doctor.

Attitudes surrounding end-of-life care have evolved significantly. Forty-five years ago, as interns and residents, we were taught never to "give up." If a patient's heart stopped, we were obligated to initiate emergency procedures: cardiac massage, intra-cardiac adrenaline injections, intubation, and manual ventilation, continuing until a senior intervened or we were physically exhausted. The patient's underlying condition—whether dementia with terminal cancer or septic shock with multi-organ failure in an elderly patient—was not a legally, ethically, or sometimes even morally relevant consideration.

Fortunately, over the decades, a shift in understanding has begun to permeate the thinking of intensivists, policymakers, and thankfully even the judiciary. This change has largely been driven by concerned families struggling to navigate the complex intersection of ICU protocols, medical ethics, law, and personal emotions. Individuals like Dr. RK Mani, an Indian intensivist dedicated to caring for the terminally ill, and Dhvani, a lawyer and co-founder of the Vidhi Centre for Legal Policy, advocating for the right to die with dignity, have been instrumental in this progress.

While active euthanasia is legal in some countries, it remains illegal in India. A patient diagnosed with a terminal illness, such as cancer, cannot legally request a lethal injection or medication to end his life, and a doctor cannot legally or ethically fulfill such a request.

The option of Active Euthanasia is illegal in India.

However, a patient, for example, a 70-year-old diagnosed with advanced pancreatic cancer that has spread to the liver and bones, can choose to execute a living will or Advance Medical Directive. This legal document allows him to specify his preferences for how he wishes to be cared for during potential decline of his health and his end-of-life care. He may choose to decline aggressive interventions like toxic chemotherapy or ICU admission when his condition worsens. This might include refusing life-sustaining treatments such as ventilators, dialysis, feeding tubes, urinary catheters, or central IV lines. While still mentally competent, he can choose to forgo some or all of these measures, acknowledging that they are unlikely to "cure" the disease or restore a "meaningful" quality of life. Instead, he can opt for "Comfort Care," recognizing that aggressive treatment at this stage often only prolongs suffering, extending life by only a short period.

***

To clarify the core of this discussion, the fundamental question is: should the medical profession utilize all available knowledge, skills, technology, and resources simply to prolong life when a return to a meaningful quality of life is improbable? Furthermore, what if both doctors and family members concur that merely extending life and suffering is not in the patient's best interest?

This crucial area is often neglected in medical curricula and training. Many doctors feel ill-equipped to discuss these sensitive issues with patients or their families. Relatives frequently request that doctors avoid mentioning "cancer," fearing it will shock and demoralize the patient. While patients have a right to know their diagnosis, in India, close relatives and caregivers often assume the role of surrogate decision-makers, asking doctors not only to conceal the diagnosis from the patient but even to fabricate an alternative diagnosis and offer false reassurances of a cure, hoping to maintain the patient's spirits.

As a doctor, ask yourself: Is prolonging life truly in the patient's best interest when recovery is unlikely and the suffering is extended?

***

Death is often perceived—and to some extent, portrayed by the media—as a medical failure. However, this perception is fundamentally flawed. Even the most powerful and seemingly invincible individuals—celebrities, scientists, royalty, and industrialists—ultimately sometimes face death, after prolonged periods of illness and suffering. No one has yet achieved immortality.

As Dr. E. Divakaran, a pioneer in palliative care from Trissur, Kerala, observes, "Death literacy is unfortunately absent or poor in India." Most people avoid discussing death with their families, who often lack the emotional capacity to handle such conversations. The typical response is denial, manifested in seeking multiple medical opinions, trying complementary or alternative therapies, and evading the crucial question: "How would you want to experience this final phase of life, and what can we do to make it as painless and peaceful as possible?"

What legal options can we recommend to patients at the end of the road?

Some of the small but significant recent legal aids we now have available, include:

1. **Withholding Treatment (WH) - This decision involves choosing not to start life support treatment. A Do-Not-Attempt-Resuscitation (DNAR) order is a considered decision, made by relatives or caregivers, to refrain from performing Cardio Pulmonary Resuscitation (CPR) in the event of an anticipated cardiac arrest in a patient for whom meaningful survival or recovery is unlikely.**
2. **Withdrawal of Treatment (WD) - This decision can be made by relatives or caregivers in the patient's best interest, to stop or discontinue ongoing life support in a terminally ill person who is no longer likely to benefit from treatment or return to a meaningful life, and where continuing treatment would cause harm and loss of dignity.**
3. **Living Will or Advanced Medical Directive (AMD) - This is a written declaration made by a person with decision-making capacity, specifying how they would like to be treated—or not treated—medically, should they lose capacity to make decisions for themselves.**

End-of-life care has improved significantly since 2023, building on the 2018 legislation, which was complex and ambiguous. However, public awareness of these provisions remains low, resulting in relatively few people creating Advance Medical Directives (AMDs) or requesting the withdrawal of life support for terminally ill loved ones.

The All India Institute of Medical Sciences (AIIMS), New Delhi, is taking a leading role by establishing an outpatient department (OPD) dedicated to raising awareness about End-of-Life Care (EOLC). These guidelines for healthcare professionals cover living wills (AMDs), powers of attorney, and Do-Not-Resuscitate (DNR) orders.

***

In many developed nations, home is the preferred place for terminally ill individuals to die. Prominent figures like U.S. President Ronald Reagan, George H.W. Bush, and Senator John McCain, as well as British celebrities and royals, including Queen Elizabeth II, chose to spend their final moments at home. In the U.S., hospital deaths from terminal illnesses have decreased from 54% fifteen years ago to around 41%, indicating a growing preference for home deaths. The UK is recognized as a leader in providing high-quality End-of-Life Care (EOLC), offering robust support to patients and families during this time.

In contrast, many urban Indians, when financially able, tend to rush ailing relatives to hospitals as death approaches. This may stem from feelings of helplessness or inadequacy in providing end-of-life care at home. Hospital or ICU admission provides a sense of having done everything possible, often masking the reality that such deaths can be lonely, overly medicalized, and impersonal, surrounded by machines and medical staff rather than loved ones in a warm, dignified setting.

***

As doctors, I urge you to engage in introspection, exercise your professional judgment, and guide your patients and their families towards a peaceful, comfortable, and dignified end-of-life experience.

I gratefully acknowledge the invaluable inputs from Dr Megha Pruthi, an exemplary palliative medicine expert and care-giver for this section.

End-of-life-care is not merely a medical protocol; it's about providing dignity and comfort to the dying patient!

LIVING WILL- SAMPLE (This document is provided as a sample of a will and should not be considered a legally binding or final version.)

ADVANCE MEDICAL DIRECTIVE (LIVING WILL) AND HEALTH CAREPOWER-OF-ATTORNEY AUTHORISATION

This Declaration on My Life is made by me (full name of the person)

....

(Date of Birth..............................; ID Document and Number.........................)

resident of (full address)

....

on (date)...at place ....

I am an adult, of sound mind and am making this 'declaration' of my own free

will, ie voluntarily and after careful consideration. If the time comes that I can no longer take part in decision making regarding my medical treatment, this 'declaration' will comprise the final expression of my wishes. It is requested that all concerned should take these wishes into account before taking any medical decision regarding my life. If at any time, I

1. Reach the stage of terminal illness and go into a coma with no reasonable expectation of regaining consciousness, or
2. Have a disease state from which I have no reasonable expectation of recovering with acceptable quality of life
3. Reach a persistent vegetative stage with no reasonable expectation of regaining significant cognitive functioning then the following steps must be taken.

I request that a panel of three doctors of appropriate expertise and experience should be constituted by the administrative head of the hospital where I am admitted for treatment. Their views should then be sought on the above. If any/all of the three situations above are confirmed then I should be deemed to have declined to receive the following life sustaining treatments as listed below. Any of these measures already started, should be removed.

1. Intravenous fluids and medications including antibiotics
2. Artificial feeding by nasogastric tube or gastrostomy
3. Dialysis
4. Artificial respiration
5. Chemotherapy
6. Cardio-pulmonary resuscitation

Other wishes : (please write by hand)

I request that this 'declaration' should be honoured by my family members and physicians as the final expression of my legal right to refuse medical or surgical treatment accepting the consequences of such refusal. This document may be informed to my regular physician..

To secure compliance with this declaration, to make medical decisions as may be required from time to time on my behalf, I hereby appoint the following as my Surrogate decision maker/s or Health Care Power-of-Attorney. S/he/they have expressed acceptance of this responsibility. I hereby vest in my attorney the power to obtain medical information, make decisions and take action on my behalf with regard to wishes expressed in this 'declaration', notwithstanding any contrary views held by any other person.

1. Name .... Signature.............................
   (Date of Birth..........; ID document and number...............
   Phone........................Email......................................)Resident
   of .... If this
   person is not available, the next two persons may be approached in the same order

2. Name ....
   .... (Date of Birth..........; ID document and number...............
   Phone........................ Email......................................)Resident
   of ....

3. Name ....
   .... (Date of Birth..........; ID document and number...............
   Phone........................ Email......................................) Resident
   of ....

In the absence of any of these authorized attorneys any member of my family will have the authority to express the wishes on my behalf regarding the above treatment.

I declare that this 'Declaration' and 'Attorney Authorization' shall remain in force during my life time unless I revoke it at any time and until notice of its revocation has been received by my attorneys.

I understand full importance of this 'Declaration' and 'Attorney Authorization'

and am fully competent to make it.

SIGNATURE

DATE........................ PLACE............................

WITNESSES:

This 'Declaration' and 'Attorney Authorization' has been signed in the presence of undersigned by .... (Name of Declarant) who is known to me and I believe that the signatory is of sound mind.

Witness I.

Name.. Signature ....

Address ....

Witness II.

Name.. Signature ....

Address ....

SIGNED BEFORE ME

APPROPRIATE AUTHORITY, STAMP

Doctor's Dilemma: Morality Vs Ethics Vs Law

" I have seen people behave badly with great morality, and I note every day that integrity has no need of rules"

Albert Camus

Morality and medicine are deeply intertwined for physicians, although ethical decisions often feel personal and subjective. We frequently rely on our conscience and individual values to determine what best serves our patients and to distinguish right from wrong. While morality has been fundamental to medical practice for centuries, moral frameworks vary across faiths, cultures, countries, and individuals, evolving with societal values. For physicians, morality centers on prioritizing the patient's best interests and ensuring no harm is done.

Medical Morals are the core beliefs that guide medical professionals on what "feels" right and what "feels" wrong in their practice.

Physicians sometimes experience conflict between their personal moral values and professional responsibilities. For example, a pregnant teenager seeking an abortion within the legal time frame has the right to the procedure. However, a physician whose religious beliefs consider terminating a pregnancy immoral, even if legally permissible and ethically acceptable within the profession, may face a moral conflict. In such cases, the physician may choose to decline the procedure based on his personal convictions.

Physicians can hold varying moral viewpoints on medical issues. Prior to the 1971 Medical Termination of Pregnancy Act, some physicians, particularly those educated in Catholic schools, resisted performing abortions on moral grounds. While societal acceptance of abortion has grown in recent decades, some physicians may still decline to perform them based on personal moral beliefs, despite their legality and ethical acceptance.

Similar moral considerations can arise in other medical situations too, such as decisions regarding passive euthanasia, administering blood transfusions to patients belonging to Jehovah's Witnesses whose religious beliefs prohibit them, prescribing medications derived from animal products. A recent example involved a devout muslim patient with pancreatitis who expressed moral concerns about taking the prescribed pancreatic enzyme supplements that are derived from the pancreas of pigs. This presented a moral dilemma for both the patient and the physician.

***

Medical Ethics, unlike personal morality, comprises a set of rules and guidelines developed by medical professionals to standardize medical practice and research. It aims to eliminate subjective and inconsistent approaches.

Ethics streamline common practices such as maintaining patient confidentiality, informing patients of all treatment options, discussing the pros and cons of recommended treatments, and obtaining informed consent before procedures like surgery. Ethics also guide us to align our practice with established guidelines and recommendations from expert medical bodies.

Consequently, any patient consulting a doctor or clinic can expect the recommended management to adhere to accepted professional standards and likely be endorsed by peers under similar circumstances.

In essence, "ethics" represents a code of conduct or set of management guidelines, recommended and agreed upon by the medical community, that competent practitioners are expected to follow for specific clinical conditions.

Medical Ethics is about following a particular set of guidelines.

Because no two patients present with identical clinical problems or circumstances, management guidelines are necessarily broad, allowing physicians to individualize their approach within those frameworks. For example, while cholecystectomy (surgical removal of the gallbladder) is generally considered the best treatment for gallbladder stones, physicians are ethically obligated to discuss all options, risks, and benefits with the patient and their family, especially if the patient is elderly, frail, has severe heart disease, and is asymptomatic. This includes the option of non-operative management, empowering the patient to make an informed decision about their care.

Medical law is the branch of law which concerns the prerogatives and responsibilities of medical professionals and the rights of the patient.

***

Medical Law dictates the mandatory practices for physicians, leaving no room for individual discretion. For example, if written informed consent from a competent adult is required before a surgical procedure, it must be obtained and documented. Failure to do so renders the physician legally liable in court, regardless of the procedure's outcome.

***

Medical morals, ethics, and law are aligned for the same purpose: the safety and "best interest of the patient."

"Medical Morals" start from an individual doctor's conscience or perspective of right and wrong. When most of us, as doctors or professionals, collectively agree on what should be the desired behavior or decision, "Medical Ethics" takes shape.

Ethics remains within the domain of our professional group or body, which we are expected to follow. Deviation from the prescribed conduct can earn us disapproval from the body or censure, but it falls short of indictment or punitive action.

If a complaint or charge against us a doctor reaches the legal arena, the court or judge must decide whether there has been a violation of the "Medical Law", whether we should be held legally liable, found guilty, and punished.

***

While the three pillars of healthcare—morals, ethics, and law—are expected to act in synergy to serve the common goal of upholding the "patient's interest," chinks or discordance are not uncommon. Here are a few examples:

Morality vs Ethics

Professor A.C. Anand, in his book *Curbside Consultation: A Glimpse into the Medical Practice in India,* recounts the case of a young resident at a prominent Indian teaching hospital caring for a young adolescent girl with acute liver failure. Her impoverished father had brought her to the emergency room in critical condition.

After exhausting all available resources, the doctor faced a difficult decision: should he inform the uneducated and financially struggling father that a liver transplant – a prohibitively expensive procedure – was the only hope for his daughter? Or should he withhold this information, guided by his own sense of "morality"?

Ultimately, the doctor chose what he considered the "ethical" course of action: disclosing and discussing all treatment options with the distraught father. Upon hearing this, the father responded, "I thought I had done everything possible for my daughter before coming here. I would have accepted her death as God's will. But now, thanks to you, I will live with the guilt of having failed to save my dying daughter!"

Ethics vs Law

Unethical medical practices, unfortunately, are not uncommon. However, many unethical decisions and actions within the medical profession remain outside the purview of the legal system and, consequently, largely unknown to the public.

A prevalent example is the immense pressure placed on wives in many Indian families to bear sons. Husbands and in-laws, particularly mothers-in-law, frequently demand a male heir.

Consider the case of a 33-year-old woman pregnant for the fourth time, already having three daughters. She faced significant social and psychological pressure, including explicit threats to her life, from her in-laws. A neighbour, a mother of three sons, secretly informed her of a doctor willing to perform sex determination via ultrasound, enabling her to decide whether to terminate the pregnancy if the child was female.

Sex determination and female feticide are illegal in India. Despite this legal prohibition, powerful societal pressures perpetuate an unethical, clandestine industry that operates largely outside the reach of the law.

In another instance, a poor farmer from a village urgently brought his frail, 80-year-old father to a nearby hospital after a sudden decline in his health. Upon evaluation in the emergency room, the elderly patient's condition rapidly worsened, necessitating resuscitation efforts. The doctor explained to the son that his father had suffered a stroke and was experiencing cardio-respiratory failure, requiring life support measures like a ventilator to survive.

The son, hesitant to make the decision alone, sought counsel from his brothers and mother. After discussion, they agreed to life support and ICU care as the thought of not doing their best for their dying father was too heavy for their hearts to bear. However, as days passed, the mounting medical expenses became an overwhelming burden. His debts spiralled, pushing him further into financial hardship. Within a week, he was bankrupt, unable to repay the loans secured by mortgaging his land. His three young children faced an uncertain future, threatened by the possibility of being sold into modern-day slavery.

The doctor, not unaware of the dire situation, continued providing the "best" possible treatment, adhering to his professional "ethics." Yet, he privately recognized the extremely low probability of the elderly man recovering or regaining a meaningful quality of life. The son, crushed by the financial strain and despair, ultimately pleaded with the doctor to turn off the ventilator and allow his father to die, believing it would prevent his family's further descent into the trap of poverty and hopelessness.

However, the son felt unable to pursue legal options or sign a Do Not Resuscitate (DNR) order due to fear of social ostracism from his community. Trapped by this impossible situation, overwhelmed by the moral conflict and financial ruin, the son saw no escape. In a tragic culmination of events, he took his own life by hanging himself, while debates surrounding legal provisions, ethics, and morality continued around him.

Morality vs Law

A 14-year-old unmarried girl was brought to a government hospital with abdominal swelling. Examination revealed a 7-month-old mobile fetus. When questioned, she acknowledged her pregnancy but begged the doctor not to inform her father, fearing for her life at the hands of her family, who were concerned about their honour.

This case presented a complex legal and moral dilemma. Obtaining a legal abortion in India for an unwed minor would be extremely challenging. Of greater concern was the very real possibility that the family, prioritizing their reputation over legal processes, might resort to killing both the girl and her unborn child.

The girl's desperate plea for help, combined with the moral and logistical complexities of the situation, has remained a deeply troubling memory for the doctor for three decades. The doctor (me!) reflects on the possible courses of action: Should he have revealed the truth to the father, attempting to reason with him and persuade him to support his daughter? Should he have admitted the girl, enlisting the support of nurses and counselors to mediate with the family? Or should he have attempted to arrange shelter for her at a Missionaries of Charity home? How could they have effectively communicated with the father and facilitated such a transfer? What could have been the social and legal repercussions of such intervention, given the limitations of working in a government-run hospital known for its insensitivity and inflexibility at the time (1992)?

***

The practice of medicine, intertwined as it is with human life and emotions, is far from simple application of knowledge and guidelines. It presents complex problems that frequently cause me to reflect deeply, constantly questioning, "What would have been the right course of action?"

Over time, I've come to understand that there are various perspectives and approaches to clinical situations, each with its own merits. There is rarely a single, "truly perfect" solution.

Actionable Insights

Dressing Appropriately

Dress to inspire confidence

My direct experience has demonstrated the profound influence of a physician's appearance on the patient-doctor dynamic. I recall Mrs. Sinha (name changed), a long-term patient with chronic hepatic issues, confiding in me about her discomfort whenever Dr. A was on duty. Her confidence waned—not due to any perceived deficiency in his medical acumen but because of his attire. He frequently wore crushed, garishly colored T-shirts, paired with jeans and informal footwear. His unkempt facial hair and noticeable body odor further compounded the issue. She once remarked, "How can I trust a physician who exhibits such sartorial negligence? If he is so casual about his own presentation, how can I expect him to exercise due diligence in my treatment?"

An individual's disposition, attitude, and character are often reflected in his attire. For a physician, his mode of dress conveys a subtle yet significant message to patients and their families, profoundly shaping perceptions and influencing trust.

In the contemporary world, characterized by rapidly evolving fashion trends and dress codes, many physicians grapple with the challenge of maintaining a professional yet contemporary appearance. Some adhere to the traditional "old-school" aesthetic—drab-coloured, loosely pleated trousers paired with standard white, regular-collared, tucked-in shirts and black shoes. While undeniably traditional, this antiquated style often prompts patients to question whether the physician's medical expertise is as outmoded as his attire.

Then there is the physician clad in poorly tailored safari suit—the archetypal "babu doctor." One can almost envision him adeptly navigating bureaucratic regulations and exploiting loopholes, while simultaneously conducting house calls for the town's elite. However, his attire tacitly suggests a professional entrenched in a bygone era, lagging behind in both contemporary medical knowledge and practice skills.

At the opposite end of the spectrum, some physicians present themselves at the hospital in attire more suited for a beach excursion—sporting flamboyant batik silk shirts, boldly striped pants, and gleaming white shoes. Their conspicuous fashion choices frequently elicit surprised reactions and generate animated discussions among patients awaiting their turn.

Young physicians sometimes arrive at the hospital attired in casual jeans, T-shirts, and athletic shoes, genuinely believing that their competence and knowledge are the sole determinants of their professional standing. However, consider the scenario of attempting to console the distraught parents of a child diagnosed with leukemia while dressed so informally. What they frequently overlook is that a physician's appearance and demeanor establish the crucial initial impression for patients and their families—knowledge and skills are evaluated subsequently.

Therefore, what constitutes the most appropriate professional presentation for a physician?

"As a patient, I expect a physician to dress smartly and formally—someone whose appearance inspires immediate confidence," states Asma Hussain, a fashion designer whose grandparents and parents have been my patients over the years. She emphasizes the essential elements: light-coloured plain or pin-striped shirts, tailored trousers (certainly not jeans), and appropriate footwear.

The white coat—or lab coat—has historically held a distinguished position within the medical profession. Worn by professionals such as myself, this knee-length garment, designed to protect underlying clothing, carries a deeper symbolic significance. For many, it represents professionalism, a visual testament to our dedication to science and the pursuit of healing.

The modern white coat, as it is recognized today, was introduced by Dr. George Armstrong, a surgeon at Montreal General Hospital and President of the Canadian Medical Association. This transition occurred in the late 19th century when physicians, seeking to distinguish themselves from charlatans and faith healers, adopted the white coat as an emblem of their scientific standing. At that time, physicians embraced this symbol, differentiating themselves from other practitioners within the medical field, such as butcher-surgeons, who wore black coats.

A doctor's appearance forms the first impression, while knowledge and skills are judged later.

The white coat is generally held in high esteem. A recent UK study demonstrated a preference among the majority of patients for their physicians to wear the white coat, prompting British hospitals to implement stringent dress codes that sometimes prohibit visible ethnic or religious symbols. This practice aims to cultivate trust and neutrality, reassuring patients who report increased confidence in professionally attired physicians.

The White Coat Ceremony (WCC), a relatively recent tradition originating at Columbia University's College of Physicians and Surgeons in 1993, symbolizes medical students' formal induction into the medical profession. The act of robing signifies their transition into a field predicated on trust and respect.

Changing Views

Despite its historical significance, the white coat, a symbol of the profession for over a century, has become a subject of contemporary debate.

"White Coat Hypertension" describes the phenomenon of elevated blood pressure readings when measured by a physician in a clinical setting (wearing a white coat) compared to readings taken at home. This discrepancy is often attributed to patient anxiety induced by the clinical environment and the white coat itself. Experienced clinicians frequently account for this effect by adjusting recorded readings or medication dosages to ensure treatment accuracy.

Furthermore, the white coat can negatively influence interactions with paediatric patients, frequently eliciting fear, crying, and resistance to physical examination. Consequently, many paediatricians have chosen to adopt more informal, colourful attire to foster rapport and facilitate cooperation during examinations.

Psychiatrists also commonly refrain from wearing the white coat, perceiving it as projecting an image of cold detachment and excessive clinical formality that could create a barrier between them and their patients. This practice reflects a conscious effort to mitigate negative stereotypes associated with mental healthcare.

A doctor's attire reflects his nature and character, influencing patients' perceptions and trust.

Considering all aspects, it is evident that attire and appearance hold substantial importance for all healthcare professionals, not solely physicians. A nurse or technician presenting in a crisp, starched uniform, complemented by a professional demeanour, immediately evokes confidence and trust. Conversely, a dishevelled or excessively flamboyant appearance can inadvertently sow seeds of doubt. This is particularly salient when interacting with apprehensive and vulnerable patients who seek visual confirmation of professionalism and trustworthiness before entrusting their well-being to their caregivers.

The core issue here does not concern a physician's or healthcare worker's personal prerogative regarding their wardrobe. Rather, it centres on cultivating a professional presentation that alleviates patient anxiety, nurtures trust, and establishes an environment conducive to comfort and compassionate care.

Medical Etiquette

We learn not in school, but life.

- Seneca the Younger

My observations have revealed that delivering effective and gratifying medical care is a considerably more intricate endeavour than it initially appears to be. It encompasses not only knowledge, skill, and ethical conduct but also a frequently neglected yet crucial element: medical etiquette. This simply denotes the appropriate decorum expected of physicians and nurses in their interactions with patients.

Regrettably, medical etiquette receives insufficient emphasis during professional training in our country, resulting in conspicuous deficiencies in professionalism. It would not be surprising if you have encountered a highly specialized physician, possessing an impressive array of credentials, who neglects basic courtesies such as offering a seat to a patient who enters the consulting room or who persists in conducting telephone conversations during a consultation. These seemingly minor oversights can significantly detract from the overall patient experience.

While adherence to etiquette may not be a matter of life or death, it undoubtedly determines whether a patient experiences comfort, feels cared for, and treated with dignity throughout the period. Over the course of my career—a sentiment echoed by many of my colleagues who have reached a similar stage of professional maturity—I have come to understand that attempting to treat patients without prioritizing their satisfaction is analogous to driving a motor vehicle without shock absorbers; while one may ultimately reach the intended destination, the journey will inevitably be arduous and uncomfortable.

***

In all fairness, it was the British—notwithstanding the frequent criticisms targeting at them—who introduced the concepts of propriety and courtesy into both general societal interactions and professional conduct. The term "etiquette," derived from the French language, conveys a similar meaning but imbues the concept with an additional element of style.

The officers of our defence forces stand as perhaps the most exemplary inheritors of this British legacy in our nation. They demonstrate punctuality, maintain impeccable dress for every occasion, and exhibit refined manners. Their displays of courtesy—towards superiors, women, colleagues, and even adversaries—are consistently measured and appropriate. However, this level of etiquette is not an inherent trait; for the vast majority, it is a product of years of rigorous training within their academies and throughout their various postings.

This British influence was once deeply embedded within Indian medical schools as well. It was so pervasive that even amidst the sweltering Indian heat, Indian doctors would habitually rub and warm their hands before examining a patient—mirroring the practice of British doctors in the frigid climate of England. Regrettably, over time, these courtesies, often referred to as "bedside manners," appear to have dissipated under the intense Indian sun.

It is noteworthy that American medical institutions are now acknowledging the importance of formally integrating medical etiquette into their training curricula. Indian doctors stand in equal, if not greater, need of such formal instruction. Perhaps it is time we turned to the officers of our defence services, who embody impeccable etiquette, to assist us in refining this critical facet of our profession.

Here are some fundamental aspects of medical etiquette that you can implement immediately:

- **Upon a patient's arrival at your clinic, rise to greet them with warmth and extend a gesture inviting them to take a seat.**
- **If you are engaged with your mobile device when a patient enters, promptly set it aside and direct your full attention to welcoming him. The patient's presence should always take precedence over any distraction.**
- **Prior to entering a colleague's clinic or examination room, particularly if he is attending to a patient, always knock. This demonstrates respect for his professional space and the patient's privacy.**
- **Maintain readily available access to a handkerchief to prevent sneezing onto either the patient or your own hands. This simple yet crucial practice contributes to maintaining hygiene and demonstrates consideration for the patient's well-being.**
- **Upon the patient's departure, extend the courtesy of opening the door for them.**

Patient's Privacy and Dignity

" Simple rule in Life: If you wouldn't like it done to you, don't do it to others"

It is echoed in many ways across time, places and cultures

" Do unto others what you would have them do unto you"

The imperative of maintaining patient confidentiality regarding disclosures and test results is frequently overlooked within the bustling atmosphere of many clinics.

During a two-week observational visit to an Indian government hospital, an American medical trainee expressed his astonishment at witnessing a young physician eliciting a patient's history from a woman in a crowded outpatient department (OPD) chamber, directly inquiring about extramarital sexual activity.

Consultation chambers in government hospitals are often characterized by a high volume of activity. Patients frequently endure extended waiting periods before being ushered into small, overcrowded rooms where overworked and often irritable physicians attend to multiple patients concurrently. In the Indian context, this typically translates to at least sixteen individuals occupying the room, as each patient typically brings at least three attendants for support and reassurance.

I have frequently observed a lack of fundamental etiquette among resident physicians undergoing subspecialty training. Within the hectic and congested OPD setting, I have witnessed them examining female patients with a blatant disregard for privacy, surrounded by unrelated onlookers. In the wards, I have observed them performing procedures, such as ascitic tap, without implementing measures to safeguard patient dignity. Another glaring infraction involves entering a patient's private room without a knock or a polite request for entry. These seemingly minor transgressions reflect negatively upon their professional conduct.

Patients in metropolitan areas, particularly those from the urban middle class, are increasingly demanding privacy and confidentiality during medical consultations. They rightfully question why unfamiliar individuals should be privy to deeply personal conversations with their physicians regarding sensitive issues such as urological symptoms or breast lumps. Ensuring that only one patient, accompanied by a single relative, is present during an examination, excluding all other individuals, should be a standard practice.

This shift in patient expectations necessitates a corresponding change in physician attitudes. Many physicians received their training in government hospitals where the sensitivities of less affluent patients were rarely prioritized. I recall an incident from my student days: an eighteen-year-old girl with a rare heart murmur was presented for diagnostic instruction. Four of us, in eagerness to learn the murmur, simultaneously placed stethoscopes on her chest, focusing solely on the clinical lesson. It was only later that I realized the tears of profound embarrassment in her eyes!

Physicians may be inclined to attribute lapses in etiquette to high workloads, staff shortages, and limited space—in essence, blaming the "system." Having worked within government hospitals throughout my career, I can attest that where there is sufficient motivation, solutions can be found.

My unwavering commitment to patient privacy, however, has not been without its challenges. During a hospital staff strike, I found myself without a designated attendant outside my consulting room. I requested a loud aggressive male attendant from the waiting area and appointed him as my temporary assistant, tasking him with managing the entry of patients. He performed this ad-hoc duty with remarkable diligence. That day remains one of the most memorable of my OPD experiences.

Since witnessing the tears of that young woman thirty-five years ago, I have been resolute in preventing a recurrence. From that pivotal moment, despite the persistent crowds and chaotic environment of the OPDs, I have consistently ensured that only one patient is present in my consulting room at any given time, while others await their turn outside.

Would you like it if you were examined from all angles infront of the curious onlooking strangers? Imagine how your patient feels. Respect their dignity by providing privacy!

Dealing with an Angry Patient

Rudeness is the weak man's imitation of strength.

-Eric Hoffer

During the nascent stages of my medical career, I consistently prioritized patient care, extending beyond the mere prescribing of medications, to help me to be genuinely attentive to his individual concerns. This approach cultivate a strong foundation of trust with my patients. Their subsequent expressions of satisfaction and gratitude reinforced my adherence to this practice.

However, the healthcare paradigm has undergone a profound transformation over the intervening years. The increasing influence of corporatization has introduced a substantial volume of administrative responsibilities, significantly limiting our capacity to allocate the requisite time and focused attention that the patient rightfully deserves. This reduction in meaningful interpersonal interaction has created a discernible deficit in both empathy and effective communication within the patient-physician relationship.

The prevailing atmosphere of trust and gratitude that once characterized these interactions has been progressively surfaced by escalating feeling of distrust, frustration, dissatisfaction, and anxiety. To effectively mend the fractured bond between physicians and patients, a thorough understanding of the fundamental causes underlying these challenging interactions becomes paramount.

Based on my extensive clinical experience, ineffective communication constitutes a primary cause contributing to the distress and animosity experienced by patients and their families toward their physicians.

I have observed this frustration manifest as a consequence of several contributing factors:

1. **Protracted Waiting Periods:** Extended waiting time can amplify a patient's pre-existing anxiety and generate a sense of being undervalued and disrespected by the healthcare system.

2. **Suboptimal Facilities or Insufficient Staffing:** If patients perceive that a healthcare facility is inadequately maintained or operates with insufficient staffing, they are likely to experience feelings of disrespect and neglect, further eroding trust in the institution and its personnel.

3. **Inadequate Explanation of Procedures and Potential Complications:** When physicians do not allocate sufficient time to comprehensively explain the potential risks and benefits associated with a proposed medical procedure, patients experience feelings of unpreparedness, heightened anxiety, and a diminished sense of control over their own healthcare journey.

4. **Difficulty in Accepting Unfavourable Outcomes:** When the results of a medical intervention do not align with the patient's expectations, it can precipitate feelings of anger, frustration, and disappointment directed toward the healthcare providers involved.

5. **Delayed or Inadequate Disclosure of Adverse Outcomes:** If patients are not promptly and transparently informed about adverse outcomes or unexpected complications, they experience feelings of betrayal, mistrust, and a sense of having been misled by their healthcare providers.

6. **A Perceived Lack of Empathy or Compassion:** When healthcare providers fail to demonstrate empathy and compassion in their interactions with patients, the latter may perceive that their concerns are being dismissed, trivialized, or not taken with due seriousness, further damaging the therapeutic alliance.

Here is what NOT to do when dealing with an angry patient:

1. **Acknowledge and legitimize the anger. Directly address the patient's emotion to de-escalate the situation. Show them you recognize and understand his feelings; legitimising it often helps to gain that patient's acceptance . Words such as " I can understand how you must be feeling right now; I would have felt quite the same in your situation", can help diffuse anger**
2. **Wait for receptiveness before explaining: If a patient is angry and unreceptive, postpone explanations until they have calmed down and are more open to discussion.**
3. **Maintain composure and avoid counter-blame: During tense moments, remain calm and professional. Refrain from counter-blaming, as this will worsen the conflict and damage the doctor-patient relationship.**
4. **Address the patient directly: Take responsibility for addressing the situation personally. Avoid delegating the task to someone else, as this can make the patient feel dismissed and undervalued.**

Instead, I recommend you do this:

1. **Acknowledge and explain delays: If a patient has experienced a long wait, directly acknowledge the delay and provide a clear explanation. For instance, say, " I am sorry that you have had to wait long.; it must have been exhausting. We've had a particularly busy morning with several patients requiring additional / emergency attention. Thanks to your understanding, we could attend to the needy on time." This validates their experience and makes them feel they have done a good deed as well.**
2. **Practice active listening: When a patient is expressing his concerns, listen attentively without interrupting. Demonstrate empathy and acknowledge his feelings. This fosters trust and strengthens the patient-doctor relationship.**
3. **Communicate clearly and provide context: Clear explanations can alleviate a patient's sense of helplessness. Provide context and answer his questions to help him feel informed and less frustrated. This demonstrates your commitment to transparent communication and patient's well-being.**
4. **Address financial concerns and offer support: Inquire about patients' financial concerns and, when appropriate, connect them with relevant social organizations or resources that can provide assistance. This demonstrates your commitment to supporting him beyond his medical needs.**

***

Consistent and ongoing communication training for all staff members is paramount for cultivating effective communication skills within the healthcare setting. Ensure that your team fully comprehends the significance of clear, empathetic, and efficient interactions with patients and their families. This training should encompass various communication techniques, including active listening, empathetic responding, and clear articulation of medical information.

Furthermore, prioritizing your own well-being is essential for effectively managing stressful patient interactions. By integrating self-care strategies such as mindfulness meditation, regular physical exercise, proper nutritional intake, and sufficient sleep, you can mitigate the risk of burnout and enhance your capacity to manage interactions with anxious or distressed patients. Investing in your own well-being ultimately translates to improved patient care and a more positive clinical environment.

Effective communication serves as the cornerstone for establishing trust and fostering mutual understanding with patients. Demonstrating empathy, practicing active listening techniques, and providing clear, comprehensive information are fundamental to this process. These practices will not only contribute to reducing patient anxiety but also prevent misunderstandings that can potentially escalate into frustration, dissatisfaction, or even conflict.

Remember, your goal is to always maintain a positive doctor-patient relationship.

How Best to Deliver Bad News

"What stands in the way is the way"

Marcus Aurelius

As Dr. Elly Hann, a specialist in end-of-life care programs, astutely observes, while the content of distressing news remains immutable, the manner of its delivery can significantly influence its impact, rendering it either a profoundly traumatic experience or a more manageable burden. This principle, it is worth noting, extends beyond the realm of medical diagnoses but applies equally to any form of unwelcome information, such as job loss, academic failure, or the dissolution of a cherished relationship.

Through experience and reflection, I have come to the understanding that adverse news, regardless of its severity, should be communicated openly rather than concealed. Transparency affords the recipient the opportunity to engage in effective coping strategies and establish realistic expectations for the future. Contemporary research has challenged the long-held assumption that imparting bad news inevitably extinguishes hope and consigns individuals to a state of irreversible despair. This, however, is contingent upon the news being conveyed with appropriate care, empathy, and sensitivity.

The currently accepted methodology for delivering difficult news is surprisingly pragmatic and possesses universal applicability in various life contexts. There are six essential components, and steps to navigate such challenging situations with greater confidence and compassion.

Let us now examine each of these steps in greater detail:

Step 1: Prepare the atmosphere for delivering bad news.

Step 2: Be aware of what the receiver already knows.

Step 3: Be aware of what the receiver wants to know.

Step 4: Gently deliver the bad news.

Step 5: Accept the reaction which the bad news evokes

Step 6: Re-assure them of your availability and support.

Step 1: Establishing the Context. Prior to conveying any unwelcome information, it is crucial to dedicate time to thoughtful preparation. Ensure that you have verified the pertinent facts and established an appropriate environment—one that affords privacy, uninterrupted time, and the presence of any necessary support persons. Consider the gravity of delivering a diagnosis as serious as cancer; such news cannot be effectively communicated amidst the distractions of ringing mobile phones, within a crowded and chaotic room, or hastily in a hallway while rushing to other commitments. It is worth noting that similar considerations apply when discussing disappointing examination results with a son or navigating a difficult conversation about a relationship dissolution with a partner. Investing time in preparation establishes a foundation for a more compassionate and sensitive exchange.

Step 2: Ascertaining Existing Knowledge. Before imparting any news, take a moment to understand the recipient's current level of awareness or any pre-existing suspicions they may harbor. For instance, a patient might already suspect the diagnosis and may be seeking confirmation. By clarifying his existing understanding, you can circumvent potential confusion and tailor your communication to the specific context.

Step 3: Gauging the Recipient's Desire for Information. Not all individuals are equally prepared to confront the full extent of a difficult truth, and it is therefore essential to assess his willingness to receive details. For example, within certain Asian cultural contexts, an elderly woman might prefer not to hear about her cancer, delegating the responsibility of receiving and processing this information, as well as making subsequent decisions, to her eldest son. In such instances, it is imperative to respect her wishes and cultural preferences.

Step 4: Communicating the Information Directly. When delivering difficult news, it is essential to be both direct and compassionate. Initiate the conversation with carefully chosen warning cues, such as, "The results have returned. I regret to inform you that the news is not favorable," or, "I need to discuss a serious matter with you; unfortunately, it is not positive." Once you have adequately prepared the recipient, articulate the news concisely, clearly, and without undue emotional embellishment. Subsequently, pause—allow them adequate time to process the information they have just received. Permit the recipient to engage in the necessary emotional processing. It is important to remember that, at this stage, non-verbal communication can often convey more profound meaning than spoken words. A simple yet reassuring gesture, such as placing a hand gently on their shoulder, can communicate empathy far more effectively than a lengthy explanation that they may not be emotionally prepared to receive. Resume speaking only after they have had the opportunity to respond.

Step 5: Addressing the Elicited Emotional Responses. Recognize that the emotional responses following the receipt of bad news can vary widely, encompassing anger, guilt, sadness, or even a sense of numbness. During this critical denial period, it is paramount to adopt the role of an active and empathetic listener. Allow the recipient's verbal expressions of emotion to unfold naturally and without interruption. Your role is not to immediately resolve or "fix" their feelings but rather to create a safe and supportive space for their expression. Simply listen attentively, without interrupting, and offer support through your presence and demonstrable understanding.

Step 6: Providing Follow-Up and Reassurance. Whether the difficult news concerns a medical diagnosis or the termination of a significant relationship, the associated pain can be profound and lasting. However, even within such challenging circumstances, you can provide valuable support by encouraging a peaceful and constructive resolution, free from animosity or hostility. Reassuring the recipient that they will not have to navigate this difficult period alone is essential for empowering them to move forward with resilience and strength.

***

Let us endeavor to collaboratively mitigate the impact of distressing news, regardless of whether it is delivered within the confines of our clinics, the privacy of our homes, or the professional setting of our offices. By approaching these sensitive moments with genuine care, empathy, and a commitment to clear and compassionate communication, we, as physicians, can significantly alleviate the burden experienced by those receiving unwelcome information and facilitate a more supportive and humane experience.

Doctor Troubles

Burnout!

Life is not a problem to be solved, but a reality to be experienced.
- Soren Kierkegaard

There are two primary factors contributing to suboptimal professional achievement. While indolence certainly plays a role, the other, somewhat paradoxical, factor is its antithesis—excessive work.

Extended working hours are a prevalent phenomenon globally. The Japanese were the first to formally recognize this phenomenon, coining the term "Karoshi," literally translating to "death by overwork."

Karoshi, or the K-Syndrome, describes the extreme repercussions of chronic overwork, frequently affecting otherwise healthy individuals, often young adults in their twenties or thirties, who consistently work exceeding 100 hours of overtime per week and subsequently succumb to sudden death attributed to "exhaustion."

Japanese individuals, particularly those within the medical profession, are renowned for their capacity to endure exceptionally long working hours.

In the post-World War II era, as Japan embarked on its extensive reconstruction efforts, prevailing circumstances and deeply ingrained cultural values fostered a strong emphasis on diligent labor. Increased work translated to greater financial remuneration, elevated social status, and perhaps most significantly, an enhanced sense of self-worth, pushing many individuals into the fold of workaholism. Consequently, young individuals began working exceptionally long hours, sacrificing sleep, and setting ambitious, often unattainable, targets for themselves.

One of the earliest documented cases involved a young Japanese worker who routinely worked 15-hour days and endured a grueling 4-hour daily commute. In another tragic instance, a 24-year-old Japanese woman tragically committed suicide after accumulating 100 hours of overtime within a single month.

This modern affliction of burnout is no longer confined to Japan; it is now increasingly affecting individuals in India as well.

Physicians, in particular, experience a profound emotional toll, with their minds and spirits often burdened by the anxiety, trauma, and anguish inherent in their profession.

The medical career path is often characterized by significant anxiety, depression, and stress from its very inception—through rigorous undergraduate program, internship, the uncertainty and arduousness of securing a postgraduate position, demanding preparation for and examinations, and the relentless pressure of cut-throat competition. This demanding process consumes anywhere from six to fourteen years of an individual's life. Sleep deprivation is a common experience during residency.

Observing young Indian professionals in metropolitan cities toiling relentlessly in offices day and night, adhering to schedules comparable to their Japanese counterparts, with limited sleep, minimal vacation time, and few opportunities for leisure activities, I am convinced that Karoshi is establishing a foothold within the India.

***

It is therefore not surprising that medical students, trainees, and practicing physicians exhibit some of the highest rates of suicide when compared to other professional groups. Burnout has devastating consequences, claiming the lives not only of individuals engaged in strenuous physical labor, such as agricultural workers or rickshaw pullers enduring harsh environmental conditions, as has long been recognized, but also of young white- and blue-collar office workers taking on the pressures of fast-paced metropolitan environments.

Data from the Indian Medical Association in Pune indicates that Indian physicians, in particular, experience significantly reduced lifespans, with mortality occurring a decade earlier, between the ages of 50 and 59, compared to the national average of approximately 70 years. Comparable findings of premature mortality among physicians relative to the general population have been documented in Poland, Japan, and numerous other nations.

Among a cohort of 282 Indian physicians studied, of whom 87% were male, the primary causes of death were identified as (1) cardiovascular diseases (27%), (2) malignant neoplasms (cancers) (25%), (3) infectious diseases (2%), and (4) suicide (1%).

Certain medical specialties appear to be associated with more adverse outcomes than others. Physicians practicing in Emergency Medicine and Anesthesiology tend to exhibit shorter lifespans compared to general practitioners and ophthalmologists, who generally experience greater longevity.

***

Despite the potential reluctance of parents, educators, and employers to acknowledge it, a growing body of evidence is pointing its finger on the association between excessive work and significant detriments to health and well-being, as well as diminished performance outcomes.

A compelling study published in the *American Journal of Epidemiology* examined a cohort of 2,000 British civil servants, who underwent cognitive assessments at two distinct time points: initially in 1999 and subsequently five years later. At the conclusion of this five-year period, researchers observed that participants who consistently worked in excess of 55 hours per week demonstrated diminished performance on tests evaluating vocabulary, reasoning abilities, emotional state, sleep patterns, and health-risk behaviors compared with their counterparts who maintained a 40-hour workweek.

Prolonged working hours have been consistently linked to a constellation of physiological and psychological consequences, including cardiovascular and immunological responses, reduced sleep duration, the adoption of unhealthy lifestyle choices, and a range of adverse health outcomes, encompassing cardiovascular disease, type 2 diabetes, subjective health complaints, persistent fatigue, and clinical depression.

Furthermore, chronic overwork during midlife may significantly elevate the risk of cognitive decline and the subsequent development of dementia in later life.

The combination of extended, unpredictable working hours and heightened stress levels also exerts a detrimental impact on family life, contributing to elevated rates of marital dissolution.

***

For several months, I have been reflecting on a recent shift in my own cognitive and emotional landscape. I have observed a disconcerting increase in forgetfulness regarding names and dates, and a transformation of my previously accommodating and nurturing disposition into one characterized by irritability and impatience.

Upon careful introspection, I have recognized that since embarking on my career as a physician, I have dedicated an excessive amount of time—approximately 90 to 100 hours per week—to clinical practice and professional conferences. Consequently, I have progressively distanced myself from activities that once provided me with enjoyment and rejuvenation, such as reading fiction, listening to music, engaging in leisure travel, and maintaining social connections with family and friends.

Could this be indicative of what is commonly termed a "mid-life crisis"? I am not sure.

To gain a more comprehensive understanding of this phenomenon, let us consider the correlation between a nation's overall happiness levels and the average working hours of its citizenry. Denmark, which consistently tops the World Health Organization's Happiness Index among 147 countries, also boasts one of the shortest average workweeks, averaging just 37 hours. This observation underscores a discernible trend: as average working hours increase within a population, the levels of happiness decrease correspondingly.

Only recently have health scientists and healthcare administrators begun to fully appreciate the urgent necessity of regulating and reducing working hours within the medical profession. Such adjustments not only contribute to a reduction in medical errors during treatment but also foster improved doctor-patient relationships, enhance patient satisfaction, and facilitate the establishment of a more stable work-life balance for healthcare professionals, affording them valuable time for personal pursuits and meaningful engagement with family and friends.

From an intuitive perspective, maintaining optimal physiological function necessitates achieving a delicate equilibrium concerning the demands placed upon the body. Insufficient physical or mental activity can lead to stagnation and lethargy, while excessive exertion can culminate in burnout and exhaustion.

Consequently, many within the medical profession, particularly surgeons, have begun to acknowledge the importance of maintaining physical fitness, preserving their psychomotor skills, and sustaining long-term professional productivity. To this end, many have adopted regular exercise regimens encompassing activities such as cycling, running, structured gym workouts, and yoga. Within urban India, some younger physicians are focusing on training for marathon events, dedicating at least one day per week to activities such as golf or tennis, or embarking on periodic trekking excursions to maintain both mental and physical well-being.

Have you begun to prioritize your own well-being? If not, what is preventing you from doing so?

Burnout at work can take a significant toll on psychological and physiological well-being, and its time to address it with a holistic approach.

Health Hazards

If you're serious about changing your life, you'll find a way. If you're not, you'll find an excuse.

-Jen Sincero

Healthcare professionals stand as the vanguard against disease, dedicating their lives to the well-being of others. However, in this pursuit of healing, they frequently encounter a multitude of occupational hazards that jeopardize their own health and well-being. From exposure to infectious pathogens to the pervasive influence of psychosocial stress, the occupational risks inherent in the medical field are both diverse and substantial.

The principal health hazards confronting healthcare workers can be categorized as follows:

Infectious Diseases: The recent COVID-19 pandemic serves as a stark reminder of this risk. It tragically claimed claiming the lives of an estimated 1,600 physicians in India alone. The World Health Organization estimates that between 80,000 and 180,000 healthcare workers worldwide may have succumbed to the virus during the 2020-2021 pandemic. A similar narrative unfolds with other infectious diseases, such as tuberculosis, with pulmonary specialists and otolaryngologists facing a high risk of contracting virulent and drug-resistant strains. Exposure to viral infections such as hepatitis B and C, and HIV also poses a significant threat. The tragic demise of the renowned Romantic English poet, Dr.

John Keats, in 1821 from tuberculosis contracted while caring for his ailing brother serves as a poignant historical example.

Ergonomic Hazards: These hazards arise from repetitive tasks that precipitate musculoskeletal disorders, including strains, sprains, back pain, and cervical discomfort. Activities such as lifting and transferring patients, prolonged periods of standing or bending, and similar physical demands can contribute to these conditions. Neurosurgeons and cardiac surgeons, who frequently perform lengthy surgical procedures requiring extended periods of standing, sustained neck flexion, and meticulous observation through microscopes, are particularly susceptible to back pain, neck pain, varicose veins, and hand stiffness. Gastroenterologists, who maintain awkward head and neck positions while observing endoscopy screens and manipulating controls, commonly experience cervical spondylosis and digital stiffness.

Chemical Hazards: Exposure to lasers, chemical agents, cleansing and disinfecting solutions, and the risk of needlestick injuries constitute additional hazards faced by healthcare personnel. Interestingly, certain aspects of these hazards have become somewhat romanticized over time. The narrative of the esteemed American surgeon Dr. William Stewart Halsted (1852-1922), credited with performing the first mastectomy and cholecystectomy (the latter on his own mother), provides a compelling example. During his tenure at Johns Hopkins Hospital, one of his operating room nurses developed an allergic reaction to mercuric chloride, a prevalent antiseptic used for sterilizing hands and equipment. In 1899, Dr. Halsted, known for his innovative approaches, contacted the Goodyear Rubber Company, renowned for its expertise in rubber technology, and commissioned the creation of thin rubber gloves to protect the nurse from the chemical irritant, enabling her to continue her professional duties.

Radiation Hazards: These hazards are prevalent among individuals working in radiology and radiotherapy departments or utilizing fluoroscopy. Early manifestations of radiation exposure can include fatigue and lassitude. Prolonged exposure significantly elevates the risk of malignancies, bone marrow disorders, and reproductive health complications.

Psychosocial Hazards: Junior physicians, nurses, and technicians who frequently assist demanding or verbally aggressive surgeons are particularly vulnerable to experiencing stress, anxiety, and burnout. The emotional burden associated with these high-pressure environments can have enduring consequences, negatively impacting their interpersonal interactions both within and outside the professional sphere. Over time, these cumulative stressors can contribute to chronic anxiety disorders, burnout syndrome, and a diminished sense of self-efficacy.

Beyond the inherent occupational risks, healthcare workers also encounter lifestyle challenges that insidiously compromise their health:

- **Physical Inactivity:** Prolonged periods of sitting in consultation rooms or standing during surgical procedures represent significant risk factors for various health problems. Extended working hours or time spent engaged in academic pursuits further exacerbate this issue. Approximately 40% of physicians acknowledge that they lack sufficient time or opportunity to engage in regular physical exercise, contributing to weight gain and diminished physical strength and stamina.

- **Unhealthy Lifestyle Practices:** Due to suboptimal lifestyle choices, a recent study revealed that 32% of physicians were classified as overweight or obese. Furthermore, extended and irregular work shifts, particularly within clinical specialties, resulted in a substantial proportion reporting inadequate sleep.

- **Substance Use (Cigarettes & Alcohol):** Many physicians resort to alcohol consumption as a means of managing stress and smoking as a perceived stress reliever following demanding shifts in the hospital or operating theater. These behaviors can subsequently evolve into habitual patterns with deleterious health consequences.

Consequently, it is not surprising that cardiovascular disease, various forms of cancer, stress-related disorders, and suicide are disproportionately prevalent within the medical profession, contributing to reduced life expectancy. We, who so eloquently counsel patients on matters of health and well-being, often become defaulters in adhering to these very principles and find ourselves in dire need of self-care and healing.

Getting Sued!

You are built to handle the pressure that comes with your calling

The pronouncement by the Supreme Court judgement in which it found three prominent city physicians and the hospital culpable of medical negligence in the untimely death of 36-year-old Anuradha Saha, and awarded a landmark compensation of Rs 6 crore to her husband, Dr. Kunal Saha, generated a palpable sense of unease within the medical fraternity.

Anuradha Saha, a resident of the United States, was visiting her parents in Kolkata in May 1998 when she developed a dermatological condition characterized by a rash and desquamation of the skin. She sought consultation with a renowned physician, who prescribed corticosteroids in dosages and frequencies exceeding established clinical guidelines. Despite the prescribed treatment, Anuradha's condition continued to deteriorate.

During her treatment, her physician had to leave for an international trip. Despite the subsequent interventions of two other specialists within the city, her condition progressively worsened. Her husband, Dr. Kunal Saha, arranged for her transfer to a hospital in Mumbai; however, she tragically succumbed to her illness within a week.

Dr. Kunal Saha, a practicing physician in the United States, attributed his wife's demise to medical negligence and initiated legal proceedings against the three Kolkata-based physicians and the Kolkata hospital. With unwavering determination, he pursued the protracted legal battle within the Indian judicial system from his residence in the United States for a period of fifteen years, seeking to establish the culpability of the physicians and the hospital. This arduous pursuit entailed substantial personal, professional, and financial sacrifices.

This landmark Supreme Court judgment on medical negligence has established a new precedent within India.

***

In the wake of instances of medical negligence, the prospect of hospitalization can understandably induce anxiety in patients; these apprehensions are neither unique nor unfounded. Hospitals, by their very nature, are environments where accidents can occur, and the recollection or dissemination of adverse experiences within a hospital setting can contribute to a pervasive sense of unease.

The World Health Organization estimates that adverse events may occur in as many as one in 300 hospital admissions, ranking these events as the tenth leading cause of hospital mortality. These incidents account for approximately 30,000 deaths annually in the United States alone. This figure stands in stark contrast to the airline industry, widely regarded as one of the safest sectors, where the accident rate is estimated at one in one million.

Consequently, medical litigation has witnessed a substantial increase in recent years. According to Dr.R.K. Sharma, a physician who subsequently specialized in the relatively nascent field of "Legal Medicine" through formal legal training, medical lawsuits have increased fivefold in recent years.

But what factors contribute to these accidents and instances of negligence?

1. **Human Error:** Human error accounts for approximately 40% of such incidents and can manifest as seemingly simple mistakes,

such as incorrectly documenting a patient's blood type or allergies, or as more complex errors, such as selecting and performing an incorrect surgical procedure. Human error is a pervasive phenomenon inherent in any organization reliant on human personnel; however, its consequences are particularly significant within the medical field, second only to the airline industry. Factors such as the quality of recruitment, the rigor of training programs, the level of professional commitment, the well-being of staff (both professionally and personally), and the effectiveness of monitoring and supervision mechanisms play crucial roles in mitigating human error. It is readily apparent that quality can be compromised at multiple levels within these systems. While human error in medicine may not result in "mass" casualties as in aviation disasters, it can lead to a series of individual adverse events, some of which may prove fatal. Within the hospital environment, such adverse events often occur when the paths of a vulnerable patient and an overworked or inattentive healthcare provider intersect.

2. **Technical Error:** Technical errors constitute the second most common category. Despite locally implemented safeguards, malfunctions in sophisticated medical equipment within hospitals do occur. Experienced clinicians often observe that in previous eras, medical interventions, while perhaps less effective, were generally safer; conversely, contemporary medical treatments, while offering greater efficacy, also carry increased risks.

3. **Organizational Failure:** Many healthcare institutions lack robust systems for monitoring and evaluating the performance quality of all staff categories. This deficiency in organizational oversight can contribute to an increased likelihood of adverse events.

***

While instances of medical negligence undoubtedly contribute to the rise in litigation, it is improbable that physicians have suddenly become collectively negligent, life expectancy has increased in recent times. One contributing factor lies in the growing awareness and assertiveness of patients in demanding accountability from their healthcare providers.

Although a degree of societal accountability is essential to ensure that healthcare professionals are held responsible for their actions, a fivefold increase in legal disputes, which increasingly portrays physicians and hospitals as culpable parties—particularly in certain regions—suggests the presence of other contributing factors. Dr. Sharma identifies two such factors:

1. **Deficient Communication:** Inadequate communication serves as a primary catalyst for many disputes. A highly competent cardiac surgeon may meticulously perform a complex procedure, dedicating countless hours in the operating room; however, if the patient does not survive, family members may become antagonistic, frequently alleging that the surgeon did not dedicate sufficient time to explaining the procedure, its associated risks, and monitor the patient's postoperative progress. The cursory two-minute consultations that were once commonplace in government hospitals are no longer acceptable. Every patient, irrespective of their socioeconomic status or literacy level, possesses the right to be informed, to have their concerns addressed, and to be treated with respect by healthcare personnel. Physicians frequently find themselves in a challenging predicament. When a physician is tasked with seeing approximately 100 patients within a mere three-hour timeframe, realistic expectations regarding the depth and quality of each interaction must be considered. I recall an instance when a newly established government hospital in Lucknow initially struggled to attract patients. To overcome this, specialists were dispatched weekly from a nearby postgraduate institute to conduct clinics. However, when each specialist managed to consult with only 15–30 patients, providing ample time and attention to each individual, the health minister of that state at that time criticized the low patient volume, demanding that the number reach 100.

2. **A Perceived Lack of Empathy:** Physicians are frequently perceived as lacking in empathy. Patients typically seek medical consultation during periods of vulnerability, often experiencing pain and fear. The bare minimum expectation is that a physician demonstrates empathy, even if overt expressions of kindness do not come naturally. Discourteous or arrogant conduct invites

animosity, and physicians must cultivate an awareness of how their actions and demeanor might be interpreted if they were in the patient's position.

***

It is undeniable that the medical fraternity is currently experiencing a state of considerable anxiety stemming from the apprehension of litigation. The good part is that heightened awareness has, fostered increased vigilance and mindfulness among physicians and medical staff in the execution of their inherently high-risk duties. These legal cases have also prompted medical teams to develop and implement standardized checklists as a means of mitigating potentially costly errors.

The pervasive fear of litigation has, unfortunately, contributed to the practice of defensive medicine among Indian physicians. This often manifests as the ordering of a significantly greater number of diagnostic tests than many financially constrained Indian patients can afford. The underlying rationale is that if a diagnosis is not "substantiated" by objective testing, physicians may face legal repercussions should complications subsequently arise.

This practice places a substantial financial burden on patients. Unlike in developed nations where medical expenses are typically covered by insurance providers or state-funded healthcare systems, the vast majority of individuals in India finance their healthcare expenditures from their limited salaries and savings.

Fear of being sued, has made doctors order more tests, just to be extra careful, which burns a hole in the poor patients' pockets!

***

While legal action can serve as a potent reminder for healthcare professionals to maintain high standards of practice, it is crucial that judges and the legal system carefully consider the potential ramifications of their judgments.

Furthermore, hospital administrations must cultivate a heightened awareness of the prevalent causes of adverse events and actively collaborate with medical staff to develop and implement effective solutions to these persistent and complex challenges.

Being Victims of Violence

An abnormal reaction to an abnormal situation is normal behaviour.
- Victor Frank

Recurrent incidents of violence perpetrated against physicians across the nation evoke fear and frustration within the healthcare workforce, including myself, eroding our sense of dedication, empathy, and commitment to service. These acts of aggression also disturb conscientious citizens and fellow patients. The escalation of violence against physicians mirrors the broader societal trend of increasing violence. Reports of verbal abuse, threats, physical assaults involving pulling collars, punches, stabbings, the throwing of furniture, attacks with blunt objects, and even shootings are disturbingly frequent. A survey of general practitioners in England, published in the *Journal of the Royal Society of Medicine,* revealed that 73% had experienced aggression within the preceding year, with 87% expressing concerns about workplace violence.

While violent behavior is most commonly encountered in psychiatric clinics and accident and emergency departments, it can manifest in any clinical setting. The typical perpetrator is a young male, frequently under the influence of alcohol or illicit substances. In emergency departments, aggressors are often family members or companions of patients, frequently arriving in large groups. The sudden occurence of tragic event, such as a fatal accident, can impair acceptance and precipitate aggressive behavior. A significant proportion of violent incidents occur following a patient's death in a hospital or during the care by a healthcare provider, with grieving relatives often attributing the adverse outcome to perceived negligence, extended waiting times, a perceived lack of empathy on the part of some physicians, or perceived inappropriate or incorrect treatment protocols.

Vandalism is a prevalent form of violence, particularly within India, often targeting physical infrastructure such as smashing windows, damaging vehicles, and vandalizing clinics and hospitals. Violence directed towards physicians and healthcare workers in India has been a persistent issue since 2006-07 and continues to show an upward trajectory. The Indian Medical Association estimates that 75% of physicians in India have experienced either physical or verbal abuse during their careers. Alarmingly, 25% of junior physicians and trainees report feeling unsafe during their hospital duties, with female healthcare workers reporting a higher prevalence of perceived threats.

Several recent incidents warrant specific mention:

1. A horrifying incident in Prayagraj in 2015, captured on video and subsequently disseminated widely, depicted a renowned super-specialist being subjected to a brutal assault by aggrieved family members in his private hospital. CCTV footage revealed individuals forcibly dragging the physician to another room and physically assaulting him for over 15 minutes. The physician had been summoned to attend to a critically ill 80-year-old patient at 4:00 AM, who tragically passed away while the physician was en route. The physician sustained a fractured jaw and multiple other injuries as a result of the violent attack. The repercussions of this incident had a deleterious impact on the community, particularly on patients requiring urgent medical attention during non-standard hours. This doctor along with colleagues and numerous other physicians practicing in smaller hospitals and nursing homes, became reluctant to respond to calls during these hours.

2. In 2017, acts of violence and vandalism erupted at Peerless Hospital in Kolkata following the declaration of a 69-year-old patient's death upon arrival. Enraged relatives engaged in destructive behavior, damaging computer equipment and shattering glass doors, temporarily disrupting healthcare services within the hospital.

3. In 2019, aggrieved relatives of a patient physically assaulted an intern at NRS Medical College Hospital in Kolkata, inflicting a skull fracture that nearly resulted in his death. Resident physicians subsequently initiated a strike, demanding enhanced security measures during their duties within government hospitals.

4. In 2023, a 25-year-old female house surgeon, Dr. Vandana Das, was tragically stabbed to death within the emergency ward of a hospital in Kerala while attending to an intoxicated patient who had been brought in by policemen. This tragic event transpired despite the presence of police officers in close proximity at the time of the assault.

5. In 2024, a female postgraduate resident physician was brutally assaulted (raped) and murdered during the night within the seminar room of RG Kar Medical College Hospital, a government teaching institution in Kolkata. This devastating incident underscored not only the inadequacy of security provisions for junior physicians but also the urgent need for significantly enhanced safety protocols within healthcare settings.

Grief and frustration constitute legitimate emotional responses for family members, particularly in the context of the loss of a loved one. However, the attitudes and reactions of healthcare consumers—patients and their families or associates—exhibit significant variation across different segments of Indian society.

Violent reactions by patients or their relatives often highlight the following underlying issues:

1. Death is frequently perceived as an unacceptable outcome within the context of hospital care. The prevailing sentiment is often, "Given the sacrifices and expenditures we have incurred to bring our loved one to this hospital, the onus now rests entirely with the healthcare providers to effect a cure." Recovery, and even a form of "immortality," is often implicitly expected, even in the case of an 85-year-old patient with a history of cardiac events.

2. There is frequently limited acceptance of adverse outcomes. Such outcomes are often perceived as a personal failure to those who have invested time, effort, and financial resources in the patient's care.

3. Physicians are often held solely accountable and subjected to punitive actions for any unfavorable outcome. In some instances, physical assaults on physicians by groups of individuals are perceived as a form of "instant justice." While individuals from less privileged socioeconomic backgrounds may resort to violence to express their anger, those from more affluent backgrounds tend to pursue legal recourse.

Opportunistic individuals, including local criminal elements, sometimes incite violence to establish themselves as vigilante figures. Similarly, local politicians may exploit these emotionally charged situations to bolster their political support, often at the expense of individual physicians who become scapegoats.

One of the consequences of this escalating aggression has been the near-discontinuation of home visits by most general practitioners. The traditional family physician, who would readily conduct house calls upon request, has become a rarity in many areas.

Qualified physicians are now hesitant to visit patients in their homes, preferring that family members transport the patient to the relative safety of a hospital setting. While the official justification often cites the logistical challenges and limitations of providing adequate diagnostic testing and medical support for critically ill patients at home, the underlying motivation for many physicians is the avoidance of potentially volatile situations within patients' homes, where anxious relatives may make unrealistic demands and issue veiled threats should the patient's condition not improve as expected.

This trend has disproportionately affected frail and elderly individuals. Beyond the inconvenience and the limited availability of reliable ambulance services, families must also contend with the substantial financial burden associated with transporting their loved ones to hospitals for medical attention.

Consequently, should you ever encounter a medical emergency at home and desire a physician's presence with a simple phone call, be prepared for disappointment.

Physicians are increasingly cautious about administering injections to seriously ill patients at home or within clinics, fearing potential aggression from relatives should the patient's condition deteriorate. This apprehension has potentially life-threatening consequences, as critical emergency interventions, such as the administration of adrenaline for severe allergic reactions, terlipressin for esophageal variceal bleeding, and anti-epileptic medications for seizures, are often delayed until the patient reaches the hospital—a delay that can often exceed two hours and sometimes prove fatal.

Practicing physicians are more likely to adopt a conservative approach, avoiding attending to critically ill patients requiring urgent care during non-standard hours, due to the fear of repercussions if outcomes do not meet the expectations of family members. Young physicians stationed in remote, under-resourced facilities or working night shifts in large government hospitals are more likely to have a low threshold for referring patients to tertiary care centers as a form of self-preservation.

It is not without reason that physicians tend to concentrate their practices in large urban centers, exhibiting reluctance to establish practices in smaller towns and rural areas. Acts of vandalism targeting clinics and physical assaults on physicians are not uncommon in smaller communities, prompting qualified physicians to relocate to more secure environments.

Violence against physicians also receives a distorted form of endorsement through portrayals in films and television dramas. It is not uncommon to witness scenes in television serials depicting bereaved family members physically accosting physicians upon receiving unfavorable news.

However, can physicians also be held partially responsible for this escalating trend?

It can be argued that physicians sometimes exhibit rudeness, insensitivity, and a lack of genuine concern in their interactions with patients and their families, which can contribute to negative reactions. The decline in the public's perception of the medical profession as a noble and revered calling is frequently attributed to perceived avarice and, in some instances, unethical practices among some physicians. It is acknowledged that every profession has its share of unethical individuals, and the medical field is no exception.

In my experience, deficient communication skills and a lack of empathy are two critical factors that impede the development of trust and a robust doctor-patient relationship. I acknowledge that these two essential skills are often underdeveloped in young physicians, particularly those who are assigned to remote areas immediately following their graduation. Distressed and agitated family members expect physicians to respond promptly, exert their best efforts, and communicate effectively. In one instance captured on CCTV, a physician was observed sitting impassively at a desk, perhaps completing a referral form, while distraught parents witnessed their critically ill child gasping and dying. The physician's body language conveyed a complete lack of the urgency and empathy that the situation demanded.

Strangely, communication skills and empathy—the two essential qualities that a doctor needs most in the world—are conspicuously absent from the medical curriculum!

The underlying disquietude originates from several systemic issues that perpetuate the problem:

The public perception of physicians has undergone a significant transformation, evolving from that of a selfless, dedicated, and compassionate caregiver to that of a profit-oriented professional. The visibility of some physicians in high-profile social circles, their conspicuous displays of affluence through extravagant attire, luxury vehicles, international travel, and opulent lifestyles, fails to inspire confidence and respect among those from less privileged socioeconomic backgrounds.

Patients from resource-constrained backgrounds often harbor expectations of care mirroring the idealized portrayals depicted in television shows within upscale private hospitals. However, upon seeking care at government-run facilities, they are confronted with starkly contrasting realities: protracted queues, overcrowded waiting areas, extended waiting times, inadequate infrastructure, and a persistent struggle to access essential resources such as beds, diagnostic tests, medications, and appropriate care. This disparity brings about feelings of disillusionment and frustration, with junior physicians, as the initial point of contact within the healthcare system, often becoming the convenient recipients of anger and wrath.

What factors impede the ability of government-run healthcare facilities to achieve parity with their privately operated counterparts?

Substandard Infrastructure: Developed nations that provide high-quality healthcare through public systems typically allocate 8 to 16% of their gross domestic product (GDP) to healthcare infrastructure development. In contrast, India's expenditure on this crucial sector remains below 2% of GDP, placing government-run facilities at a significant disadvantage.

Systemic Mismanagement: The administration of government health services is frequently characterized by inefficiency and mismanagement, as evidenced by recent investigations conducted by the Central Bureau of Investigation (CBI) in 2024 following a tragic incident in West Bengal. Issues pertaining to staffing levels, service delivery, the quality and availability of essential supplies, as well as inadequate monitoring and accountability mechanisms, present a concerning picture. Similar systemic deficiencies likely exist in many other states.

Escalating Healthcare Costs: The cost of healthcare services is rapidly escalating, placing a significant financial strain on individuals. Healthcare expenditure is still predominantly an out-of-pocket expense for most Indians. Within a population of 1.4 billion, substantial segments of society lack the financial capacity to afford adequate healthcare on their limited incomes, while others are driven into debt when seeking treatment at expensive private facilities. Alarmingly, only approximately half of the population possesses any form of health insurance coverage.

The Expanding Private Sector: A significant portion of healthcare provision has transitioned to the private sector, driven by the government's inability to meet the growing demand for advanced medical technology, modern facilities, and elevated service standards, compounded by rising costs and a reluctance to adapt to evolving needs. Prior to 1980, the majority of healthcare services in India were delivered by government institutions. Today, the private sector caters to approximately 70% of the nation's healthcare needs. While private entities have played a role in addressing service gaps, their investments are inherently motivated by profit generation. Concurrently, healthcare demands and associated costs have risen dramatically, outpacing the financial capacity of many individuals in resource-constrained areas who continue to rely on government-provided healthcare.

The number of medical colleges within the country has increased significantly, from approximately 200, primarily government-run institutions, to over 600 today, with private institutions accounting for the majority of this expansion. The cost of medical education within these institutions has also increased considerably, thereby catering to students from more affluent backgrounds. Consequently, graduates from these private institutions, having invested substantial sums in their education, often prioritize recovering their financial outlay as expeditiously as possible. This paradigm shift has contributed to perceptible changes in the professional ethos and public perception of physicians in contemporary society.

Hospitals, both within the public and private sectors, bear the responsibility of providing a safe and secure working environment for their physicians and healthcare personnel. In the current context, this necessitates the deployment of adequately trained security personnel, the installation of comprehensive CCTV surveillance systems, the digitization of patient data, and the implementation of robust monitoring protocols for medication dispensing processes—all of which require significant financial investment. As health is a matter under state jurisdiction, each state government must ensure that these measures are effectively implemented and rigorously monitored. Unfortunately, a deficiency of political will and motivation often results in substantial shortcomings in these areas.

Resorting to violence as a means of addressing perceived physician misconduct is ultimately counterproductive; such actions are unlikely to induce positive change in unethical practitioners and may even exacerbate their indifference, while ethical and dedicated physicians, who previously went above and beyond for their patients, may become hesitant to do so for fear of reprisal.

It is imperative to recognize that empathy cannot be coerced or mandated. A safe, supportive, and conducive environment is essential for physicians to cultivate compassion and deliver optimal patient care.

To mitigate the risk of violent confrontations and effectively manage such situations should they arise, consider the following strategies:

- Cultivate and refine your capacity for empathy and compassion. Even if these qualities do not come naturally, developing them, even later in your professional trajectory, is still worth the effort. Diligently dedicate time to actively listening to both the patient and his accompanying family members. Demonstrate genuine concern for his expressed anxieties and medical issues, and when appropriate within the cultural context, approach the patient's bedside and offer a reassuring touch as a gesture of support.
- Communicate your clinical assessment and the proposed treatment plan with clarity and transparency.
- When communicating with patients and his family, frame your responses in terms of the interventions you can provide, such as administering intravenous fluids, providing pain relief medication, applying splints, or prescribing appropriate antibiotics. Unless specifically queried, refrain from emphasizing what cannot be accomplished.
- Avoid engaging in confrontational exchanges or heated arguments with an agitated group of individuals. Direct confrontation should be avoided, particularly when you are alone and unsupported. It is crucial to remember that a crowd driven by collective anger is often impervious to reason and can react violently to even minor provocations or instigations. In such volatile circumstances, discretion and prudence are paramount. It is far more prudent to seek security assistance or to address the situation collectively with colleagues.
- If patients or their family members express a desire to seek medical care at another facility, such as a more specialized or advanced center, adopt an encouraging and supportive stance. A facilitative approach is considerably more effective than exhibiting frustration or resentment at the capabilities of the current facility. An ego-driven response, characterized by attempts to assert superior expertise or imply that other institutions cannot provide better care, is highly likely to be counterproductive and potentially exacerbate the situation.

Doctors: Behind the Scenes

Why do Doctors take U-Turns on their Advice?

Medicine is a science of uncertainty and an art of probability.

-William Osler

Medical science is not a static discipline; it continually evolves, shedding outdated concepts and embracing new paradigms as novel evidence and therapeutic interventions emerge.

Consequently, physicians are trained to assimilate the constantly evolving landscape of research findings and to integrate them into clinical practice from time to time.

Indeed, medical students are frequently assessed in examinations on demonstrating a thorough understanding of the most recent advances in the medical field. Furthermore, patients, with their ready access to online information, often evaluate our competence based on how updated we seem to be with contemporary developments.

However, research scientists are known to frequently revise or even contradict their own recommendations from previous years.

For example, a recent study suggests that consuming more than three eggs per week may increase the risk of premature death. Were my grandmother alive today, I could almost hear her say, "What is new about this information? I have been telling this all along!"

Yet, throughout my four decades of medical training and practice, eggs were consistently lauded as an exceptional source of dietary protein. In fact, the medical community, governmental agencies, and poultry industry stakeholders actively promoted their consumption as an effective strategy for combating protein malnutrition.

I now find myself contemplating how a surgeon colleague of 35 years—whose customary breakfast has invariably consisted of a double-egg omelette accompanied by two slices of toasted bread—intends to reconcile this new dietary guidance with his established habits.

A similar controversy has arisen regarding blood lipids—cholesterol and triglycerides—the fatty substances that circulate within our bloodstream, coating the inner walls of our arteries. They were previously considered primary culprits for myocardial infarction (heart attacks). In a surprising reversal of prior medical understanding, these lipids have now been largely exonerated. Medications that were once widely prescribed and consumed in vast quantities to lower cholesterol levels in order to prolong lifespan are now being labled as potentially unnecessary at best and detrimental at worst.

Another example of shifting medical perspectives stems from a recent publication that challenges the widespread practice of prophylactic low-dose aspirin administration among adult males for the prevention of heart attacks. Aspirin had previously been shown to reduce platelet aggregation within the circulating blood, a mechanism that scientists hypothesized to be an initial trigger for the formation of arterial and cerebrovascular thrombi (blood clots). Following several years of widespread aspirin use for this purpose, medical researchers have now demonstrated that it offers negligible benefit and may, in fact, precipitate potentially fatal gastrointestinal bleeding in several individuals. Consequently, its use as a preventive strategy in individuals without pre-existing cardiovascular disease is now being questioned.

Vaccination, a practice widely accepted for preventing several infectious diseases and reducing mortality rates, particularly among children, has also become a subject of debate. Public perceptions have shifted significantly in recent years, with a proliferation of anti-vaccination advocacy groups. They often express strong convictions that many childhood vaccines caused harm. Against this backdrop of public skepticism, the United States recently experienced a significant outbreak of measles among children whose parents had declined vaccination.

While these newly emerging individual research studies may be valid, the same level of certainty cannot always be ascribed to the evolving medical guidelines that they support.

You may have come across the following post that was making the rounds on Facebook:

An Interesting Fact,

Before 1997, the fasting sugar limit for Diabetes was 140.

WHO put a panel to decrease it and was fixed it as 126.

All of a sudden 14% of world population became diabetic overnight.

Later in 2003, American Diabetic Association again decreased the limit to 100.

And after this 90% of Indian population became diabetic.

And you know who are the members of those panels deciding the fasting sugar limit??

They are the consultants of 7 big pharmaceutical companies in world!

So in short, it's the Pharma industry that decide if you are diabetic or not.

Be aware !

A comparable trend is seen in the management of blood pressure and cholesterol levels. While it is undeniable that meticulous control of blood glucose and blood pressure have contributed to improved health outcomes and increased longevity, it is equally true that medications for diabetes, hypertension, and cholesterol constitute a significant revenue stream for numerous pharmaceutical corporations. An increase in diagnoses directly correlates with augmented sales and profitability.

This phenomenon extends across a wide range of medical specialties, including gastroenterology and hepatology. Medications that suppress gastric acid production, known as Proton Pump Inhibitors (PPIs), represent another highly lucrative product category for the pharmaceutical industry.

Furthermore, the standard treatment protocol for Hepatitis C until recently, involving weekly injections of interferon accompanied by significant adverse effects and suboptimal cure rates, has been completely revolutionized. With the advent of highly efficacious and well-tolerated oral medications within the past few years, all existing clinical guidelines have been revised to incorporate these novel therapeutic agents. Indeed, guidelines for the management of Hepatitis B and Hepatitis C are now published and updated almost annually, often with the support or sponsorship of pharmaceutical companies.

This raises pertinent questions regarding the forces driving these changing guidelines. Who orchestrates the periodic public health alarms regarding influenza outbreaks (such as swine flu or avian influenza) and the resulting societal pressure that compels individuals experiencing even mild febrile symptoms to seek immediate medical attention and undergo specialized diagnostic blood tests—tests that are often manufactured and distributed by a single multinational corporation, sold to governments of developing nations at inflated prices? The potential interconnections between the pharmaceutical industry and the bodies responsible for formulating clinical guidelines becomes suspect, although definitively proving such connections often presents a considerable challenge.

Regardless of the underlying factors, whether they be driven by legitimate scientific advancements or influenced by other considerations, these frequent and often abrupt shifts in medical understanding create a perception of inconsistency and even incompetence among healthcare professionals, particularly when we are compelled to take back what we had advised a short while ago!

Prescription of Problems

My love is like a doctor's handwriting, it is only understood by you!

Prescriptions, while constituting a fundamental aspect of medical practice, present a unique set of challenges.

The stereotypical "doctor's prescription," characterized by illegible handwriting that could often only be deciphered by a local pharmacist, is poised to become a relic of the past.

For reasons that remain somewhat enigmatic, physicians' poor penmanship has become a subject of widespread humor and a source of numerous anecdotes. It is likely that most physicians have encountered instances where a patient has inadvertently taken the incorrect medication due to a misinterpretation of a handwritten prescription. I recall a case involving a young woman with a thyroid disorder who had been prescribed "Ciplar" to regulate her rapid heart rate; however, due to a misreading by the pharmacist, she received "Ciplin" (an antibiotic) instead, subsequently developing persistent nausea.

The Medical Council of India has now mandated that physicians provide either printed prescriptions or write them legibly in capital letters. This initiative appears to be well-intentioned and should improve the accessibility and comprehension of medical prescriptions, not only for pharmacists but also for patients themselves. This is indeed a positive development.

While enhancing the readability of prescriptions represents a significant advancement, efforts to reform prescribing practices extend beyond this measure.

Regulatory bodies have further advocated for physicians to prescribe generic medications, rather than their commercial branded names. Generic formulations, which denote the specific chemical compound—such as aspirin—are generally more affordable than their branded counterparts (e.g., Dispirin) marketed by pharmaceutical companies.

However, this practice also presents certain drawbacks.

Many pharmaceutical industry executives privately acknowledge that the quality of generic and branded medications, while officially deemed equal, may not always be precisely comparable. Discerning readers will readily understand how the quality of both generic and branded versions of the same chemical entity, manufactured and distributed by a single company, can be associated with disparate pricing structures.

When treating patients with serious medical conditions, physicians often prioritize trusted brand-name medications, notwithstanding their higher cost. Can physicians justifiably take risks, for instance, when managing a critically ill patient with typhoid fever and septic shock, by administering an antibiotic from an unfamiliar source? Furthermore, if the patient were a close relative, would one not prefer a medication from a reputable pharmaceutical company, even if it entailed a greater financial burden?

If regulations mandate the exclusive use of generic names on prescriptions, the discretion of selecting the appropriate medication would effectively shift from the physician to the pharmacist or hospital administrator. The potential motivations for a dispensing pharmacist—who does not have direct responsibility for the patient's well-being—to favor one company's medication over another require little elaboration.

Beyond the ongoing debate concerning generic versus branded medications lies another pressing issue: the prevalence of lengthy prescriptions.

As is commonly observed, medical prescriptions rarely consist of a single medication; they frequently encompass an extensive list of pharmaceuticals. Ironically, the patient may have presented with only a single symptom. This phenomenon has recently been termed the "Prescription Cascade."

Given that most medications are associated with potential side effects, physicians often prescribe additional medications to counteract these anticipated adverse reactions. A common illustration of this practice is the co-prescription of medications that reduce gastric acidity alongside pain relievers.

Most analgesics, such as aspirin, ibuprofen, diclofenac, indomethacin, and naproxen, can cause gastric irritation, leading to gastritis or gastric erosions. In fact, long-term use of these agents is associated with the development of gastric or duodenal ulcers, which, in addition to causing abdominal pain, can sometimes result in bleeding or perforation, posing a life-threatening risk. To mitigate this risk, physicians often find it more convenient, and perhaps safer, to concurrently prescribe a proton pump inhibitor (PPI), such as omeprazole, pantoprazole, or rabeprazole, which suppresses gastric acid and reduces the likelihood of developing ulcers. While most PPIs are generally well-tolerated, they significantly increase cost of treatment. For instance, aspirin for chronic back pain might cost approximately Rs 2 per day, whereas a PPI would add an additional cost of approximately Rs 5 per day. Over a one-month period, the cost of treating the back pain itself would be Rs 60, but the cost of preventing a potential adverse effect of the primary treatment would be Rs 300.

Another common example is the co-prescription of antibiotics with probiotics. Antibiotics, prescribed for bacterial infections, frequently disrupt the balance of the gut microbiota, the beneficial bacteria residing within the intestines that contribute to overall health. This disruption can manifest as antibiotic-associated diarrhoea. To counteract this, it has become standard practice to prescribe probiotics, which contain mixtures of beneficial bacteria. These probiotic supplements typically cost between Rs 30 and Rs 60 per day, sometimes exceeding the cost of the antibiotics themselves, and often require administration for a duration extending beyond the typical 5-day course of antibiotic therapy. This practice imposes a significant financial burden on patients.

Several medications, such as anti-amoebic agents and chemotherapeutic drugs, can induce nausea and vomiting. These are routinely co-prescribed with antiemetic medications to mitigate these adverse effects. This can create further complexities, as these secondary medications can themselves cause side effects, such as extrapyramidal symptoms (abnormal muscle movements), drowsiness, or galactorrhea (breast milk production), potentially generating more concern than the original side effects of the primary medication.

***

From the longstanding challenge of illegible handwriting, which poses a risk of miscommunication and medication errors, to the ongoing discourse surrounding generic versus branded pharmaceuticals and their implications for affordability, and the intricate matter of polypharmacy (the prescription of multiple medications to manage side effects), each facet of the prescribing process warrants careful deliberation and nuanced understanding. While the practice of prescribing multiple medications concurrently, often referred to as a "prescription cascade," can, in certain clinical scenarios, contribute to improved therapeutic outcomes by mitigating adverse drug reactions or addressing comorbid conditions, it also inevitably increases the financial burden on patients and introduces the potential for additional drug interactions and side effects. This necessitates a delicate balance between clinical necessity and judicious prescribing practices.

As physicians, our fundamental objective remains: the well-being of our patients. Although we are frequently subjected to criticism and public skepticism, it is an indisputable truth that our dedication to their recovery and overall health extends far beyond what is commonly perceived. Ultimately, no physician desires the loss of a patient; our endeavors, while not always perfect or without limitations, are invariably grounded in a genuine desire to provide compassionate care and facilitate healing. Perhaps, in the specific context of prescription writing, the principle of parsimony—keeping things simple and prescribing only what is absolutely necessary—is a valuable lesson worthy of consistent application.

How Doctors Really Diagnose?

Never confuse education with intelligence. You can have a master's degree and still be an idiot.

While I would refrain from asserting that physicians possess a monopoly on intellectual prowess within society, the intriguing cognitive processes we employ and the unique manner in which we arrive at clinical decisions have consistently captivated researchers. Dr. Jerome Groopman delves into this very subject with considerable insight in his book, 'How Doctors Think'.

As physicians, we tend to rely heavily on specific cognitive functions, with memory serving as a cornerstone, particularly during the initial stages of our training. From the moment we commit to pursuing a career in medicine and undertake the entrance examinations for medical school, we are expected to absorb, retain, and subsequently reproduce a vast quantity of factual information—anatomical nomenclature, physiological functions, and a plethora of intricate details. Unlike students pursuing disciplines such as engineering, management, or law, our initial training does not primarily emphasize mathematical problem-solving, creative ideation, or unconventional logical reasoning. Instead, we excel at recalling the names and characteristics of thousands of organs, tissues, cells, and pharmaceutical agents, often with remarkable precision and recall.

As we progress into the clinical phase of our training, we develop the ability to recognize recurring "patterns" of symptoms and physical signs exhibited by patients and attempt to integrate these observations into a diagnostic framework. For instance, the presentation of chest pain accompanied by diaphoresis (sweating) would strongly suggest a myocardial infarction (heart attack), while the concurrence of jaundice and anorexia (loss of appetite) would suggest the a diagnosis of hepatitis.

With increasing clinical experience, we cultivate a cognitive approach known as "probabilistic" thinking, wherein the patient's individual profile assumes greater significance than isolated symptoms. Using the example of chest pain, we recognize that this symptom in a healthy 20-year-old female is almost invariably attributable to musculoskeletal factors and rarely indicative of cardiac pathology. Conversely, in a 50-year-old overweight male with a history of smoking and hypertension, the same symptom is highly suggestive of a myocardial infarction, necessitating immediate referral to a cardiac intensive care unit.

As our careers advance, we begin to incorporate multiple facets of our patients' individual circumstances into the decision-making process. This is the stage at which we begin to synthesize the "art" of clinical judgment with the extensive body of textbook knowledge acquired during our medical education. Does the vegetable vendor, presenting with cough and fever following exposure to inclement weather, truly require a computed tomography (CT) scan of the chest, or would empirical antibiotic therapy suffice? Does a 16-year-old female student experiencing acute onset vomiting prior to her board examinations require immediate endoscopic evaluation? What if she experienced similar symptoms during a stressful examination period the previous year?

As we mature as clinicians, we transcend the role of mere repositories of facts, information, and knowledge. It is the unconscious integration of years of accumulated experience, refined by a compassionate understanding of our patients' concerns and constraints, and supplemented by a degree of clinical intuition, that ultimately guides us in making decisions that are frequently validated by subsequent tests or course.

In contemporary medical practice, interactions with patients can often be quite illuminating. I frequently encounter patients who are overly eager to receive the results of their diagnostic tests, believing that the reports themselves will provide a definitive explanation for their symptoms. I then find myself in the position of having to explain, often to their surprise, why the interpretation of diagnostic reports must be considered within the broader clinical context and are not, in isolation, sufficient for establishing a diagnosis. There is no test that helps diagnose migraine or anxiety!

**Good clinical decision making,
like good wine, matures over time.
Knowledge alone does not make a good
doctor; the flavour matters too!**

"How Can You Fall Sick? You are a Doctor!"

Sickness and death are unavoidable in life. To experience illness is not itself misfortune, but to be defeated by illness is.

It is a paradox that despite our extensive medical knowledge concerning the human body, its myriad pathologies, and available therapeutic interventions, physicians cannot escape illness and death. Our health status and life expectancy are not demonstrably different from those of the general population. The salient distinction lies in the fact that physicians frequently elect to forgo the arduous and often invasive treatments that they routinely recommend for their patients.

In a compelling article entitled "How Doctors Choose to Die," Dr. Ken Murray elucidates the tendency among physicians to eschew "advanced" and "intensive" therapeutic modalities for themselves.

We are statistically more likely to decline chemotherapy when diagnosed with advanced neoplastic disease, choosing instead to prioritize the remaining quality of our lives and spend valuable time within the familiar comfort of our homes. We may also refuse aggressive end-of-life interventions. These decisions are likely informed by our direct observations of the distressing adverse effects and often limited clinical efficacy of such treatments in our patients.

Despite generally having unimpeded access to any medical intervention we might require, we frequently choose to decline them. We have witnessed the potential outcomes firsthand. We possess sufficient understanding of the process of dying to comprehend the most prevalent human anxieties surrounding it: the fear of experiencing death in a state of intractable pain and in complete isolation. We are acutely cognizant of the inherent limitations of contemporary medical practice. Almost all of us have observed instances of "futile care" being administered. The patient undergoes invasive surgical procedures, is subjected to a multitude of indwelling catheters and tubes, is connected to complex life-support systems, and receives a vast array of pharmacological agents, often without achieving any meaningful clinical improvement.

In a certain respect, physicians might be accused of practicing double standards, applying one set of recommendations to patients while adopting a different one for himself. However, the crucial mediating factor in these situations is often the expectations and desires of family members. When a patient's condition deteriorates precipitously, even if they are advanced in age (for example, 85 years old) and known to be afflicted with a terminal illness, the prevailing sentiment expressed by their relatives is typically, "Do everything humanly possible."

In our current societal climate, characterized by a proclivity for assigning blame, identifying scapegoats, and pursuing litigation, physicians often feel professionally and legally obligated to pursue all conceivable treatment options. Family members, many of whom may have traveled considerable distances to be present, often derive solace from the feeling that they have exhausted every available resource in the care of their loved one, thus freeing themselves from potential feelings of guilt associated with perceived inaction.

It is precisely this fear of subsequent guilt that frequently compels family members to subject their loved ones to dehumanizing and often futile end-of-life treatments: surrounded by unfamiliar medical personnel within the sterile environment of an intensive care unit, connected to complex and often alarming machinery, their bodies subjected to multiple invasive procedures, and often deprived of the comforting presence of familiar and loving faces during their final moments.

There is good reason to accept the adage, "The road to hell is paved with good intentions."

Do Doctors Go To Doctors?

The relationship between patients and physicians is becoming increasingly rough. Media outlets, both traditional and social, frequently publicize incidents of physicians being assaulted by irate family members. This phenomenon of physician-bashing appears to have evolved into a contemporary outlet for collective frustration, analogous to a modern form of public shaming or vigilantism.

Today, I wish to direct attention to the opposite end of the patient-physician spectrum: the potential detriments of excessive familiarity and friendship within this professional relationship. These dynamics, while often less overtly disruptive, can be equally detrimental, albeit in a more insidious manner.

I once encountered a rather unique patient. She was a senior physician and academician hailing from a major city. What was particularly striking was the fact that she had scheduled an online consultation without disclosing her own medical background to me, nor did she request any preferential treatment or fee waiver.

As our consultation progressed, I discovered that she had been grappling with a constellation of health issues for many years, including decades of indigestion attributed to wheat sensitivity, several years of arthritis, and significant obesity, among others. Towards the conclusion of our session, as I began to suggest the names of several respected gastroenterologists in her city for further consultation, she said with a grimace, "I've consulted with them on numerous occasions… that's precisely why I sought your opinion here, where I am unknown."

Her statement resonated deeply. Here was an individual who had become weary of the excessive familiarity that had developed with her regular physicians—those who would readily answer her calls at inconvenient hours and offer medical advice over the telephone.

She confided that whenever she mentioned her symptoms during informal social gatherings, such as Diwali dinners with physician acquaintances, her concerns were often dismissed with cursory, temporary prescriptions.

This over-familiarity had ultimately proven detrimental to her health. Her recurring episodes of loose stools had been "managed" via telephonic consultations with short courses of antibiotics for a period of four years before a physician outside her social circle finally diagnosed her with celiac disease. Similarly, her debilitating arthritis had been neglected for several years until another physician, practicing in a different locality, conducted a thorough physical examination, ordered appropriate diagnostic investigations, and initiated a suitable treatment plan.

Regarding her weight, none of her "doctor-dosts" (physician friends) felt comfortable broaching the topic of dietary modification or portion control during social events. Unsurprisingly, her weight had gradually increased to nearly 100 kilograms. This situation served as a stark reminder of how excessive familiarity, even within professional contexts, can sometimes have more deleterious consequences than beneficial ones.

A prevalent tendency exists among many individuals to seek friendships with physicians, often with the expectation that they will be readily available to answer calls and provide medical advice on the corridor. I cannot recall attending a single social gathering without at least one guest requesting my personal contact information. Interestingly, I have never observed anyone making similar requests of bureaucrats, government ministers, or law enforcement officers.

This very phenomenon of excessive familiarity with physicians—those casual telephonic consultations and informal medical discussions at social events—had ultimately proven detrimental to this particular patient. Clinical judgment cannot maintain its necessary acuity and precision when it is clouded by undue familiarity and relegated to brief phone calls or amidst informal conversations at social gatherings. Patients must recognize the potential risks they assume when seeking medical advice in such a casual and informal manner for the sake of convenience.

When a friend seeks your medical help, try to see beyond friendship and diagnose them with the same professionalism and thoroughness you would offer any other patient.

Cruelty in Doctors: Does it Matter if a Doctor is Cruel to Animals?

"The greatness of a nation can be judged by the way its animals are treated"

Mahatma Gandhi

The recent case of two medical students sadistically throwing a puppy from a fifth-floor terrace, filming the act, and sharing it online with a disturbing sense of accomplishment was deeply troubling to all who saw it. The blatant cruelty is compounded by the fact that these individuals were aspiring doctors.

This incident should serve as a stark warning to medical policymakers and administrators. Our current focus on objective, knowledge-based assessments for medical students and doctors has created a significant blind spot.

Is medical knowledge and a degree sufficient in the making of a modern doctor, or whether empathy and kindness be considered too? Ponder over it.

While the importance of humane qualities in doctors is widely acknowledged, the challenge lies in reliably assessing and measuring them. Management experts recognize that organizational performance depends on more than just intelligence, leading to a shift in focus from IQ to EQ. While other sectors have adopted this understanding, medical recruitment and promotion remain largely archaic, relying heavily on MCQ scores, publications, and citations.

Historically, links between animal cruelty and violence against humans are well-documented. Serial killers like Albert DeSalvo and Dennis Rader exhibited early patterns of animal abuse. Studies have even shown a strong correlation between animal cruelty and sexual homicide.

Cruelty to animals is not a minor flaw but a sign of deeper mental disturbance. Research indicates that those who abuse animals often escalate to harming humans. Such acts should be red flags, suggesting a potential for abuse within families and society.

Medical schools and regulatory bodies must re-emphasize the importance of kindness and empathy in doctors. They need to develop reliable methods for evaluating and measuring these qualities in aspiring medical professionals and integrate them into assessment systems. Without these virtues, the medical profession risks becoming a mere business, devoid of the nobility, empathy, and respect it once commanded.

Princely Patients

What's in the Menu?

You have your way. I have my way. As for the right way, the correct way,and the only way, it does not exist.

-Friedrich Nietzsche

A patient's comfort level with a particular physician often hinges on the congruence between their respective attitudes and expectations. When a harmonious alignment exists, the patient is more likely to experience a sense of ease and trust in the physician's care.

In previous eras, physicians frequently adopted a "paternalistic" approach, wherein we unilaterally determined the most appropriate course of action for the patient. We would prescribe a specific treatment regimen, and the patient would typically adhere to it without question. Assuming a quasi-parental role, we would assess the patient's needs, tolerance for various interventions, and financial capacity, and then direct them accordingly. Many patients continue to prefer this straightforward approach, often asking directly, "Doctor, please advise me on what I should do."

This paternalistic model was more fitting in a historical context where therapeutic options were limited or nonexistent, and the physician-patient relationship was largely predicated on implicit trust and deference. However, given the proliferation of treatment modalities available today and the increasingly informed expectations of patients, this approach is becoming progressively obsolete.

In contemporary medical practice, the prevailing expectation is for physicians to adopt a "cafeteria approach." This entails presenting all viable treatment options to the patient, clearly delineating the associated risks and benefits of each, and facilitating their informed selection from this "menu" of choices. For instance, when discussing the management of coronary artery disease, I might thoroughly explain the potential risks and benefits of three distinct options: continued medical management with pharmacotherapy, percutaneous coronary intervention (angioplasty), or coronary artery bypass graft surgery.

Each of these options carries its own set of advantages and disadvantages, contingent on factors such as the severity of the disease, the patient's age and overall health status, and his ability to tolerate invasive procedures. I also prioritize open and honest communication regarding the financial implications of each treatment strategy and clearly articulate my own level of expertise in performing or managing these interventions, empowering the patient to make a well-informed decision. In this model, the patient effectively "directs" the physician regarding the preferred course of action.

While physicians often seek a definitive, quantifiable answer to present to patients, such clarity is not always attainable. Consider, for example, a 60-year-old man contemplating coronary artery bypass surgery. How does one accurately weigh the 2% risk of perioperative mortality against an 85% probability of survival over a five-year period if the surgery is successful, particularly when his daughter's wedding is scheduled in just six months?

The responsibility for decisions with potentially adverse outcomes is consequently shifting from physicians to the patients themselves. As societal litigiousness increases, compelling us to practice defensively, we find it more expedient, albeit more time-consuming, to present relevant facts and statistical data and allow the patient to determine their own course. However, given the financial incentives associated with surgical procedures and interventions, we do, at times, consciously or unconsciously, inject our own biases into these discussions. Have you not encountered a laparoscopic surgeon who subtly emphasizes the "slight" but tangible risk of malignancy developing in the gallbladder if asymptomatic gallstones are not surgically removed? Or have you not heard a cardiologist recount an anecdote about a patient who declined angioplasty and subsequently experienced a cardiac event?

Doctor Hopping, Medical Shopping

Don't trust blindly …… ..but
Not being able to trust others is a big symptom of not being able to trust yourself

The distinction between seeking a "second opinion" and engaging in what is commonly termed "doctor hopping" or "medical shopping" is often indistinct and subject to interpretation.

A "second opinion" entails seeking consultation from another medical professional to corroborate or validate a diagnosis or treatment plan provided by the initial physician. This practice can be a valuable step in ensuring diagnostic accuracy and optimizing treatment strategies. Most individuals, operating with sound judgment, would not typically seek a second opinion for a common, self-limiting ailment such as a mild upper respiratory tract infection. Conversely, if the initial diagnosis is of a serious nature, such as a malignancy (cancer), or if the recommended treatment is invasive, expensive, or carries significant risks, such as cardiac surgery, it is entirely reasonable and understandable for a patient to seek confirmation or endorsement from another expert in the relevant medical specialty.

In fact, ethical and conscientious physicians and surgeons frequently encourage their patients to obtain a second opinion, particularly when delivering unfavorable diagnoses. This practice serves to reinforce the validity of the diagnosis and can facilitate greater patient acceptance of the recommended treatment plan, thereby enhancing adherence and improving outcomes. This process allows patients to return to their original physician with increased confidence and motivation to undergo the necessary interventions.

Seeking a second opinion can strengthen the patient's confidence in your diagnosis and prepare them to approach the recommended treatment with greater resolve.

The diagnosis of malignancy is unequivocally one such circumstance. It frequently arrives as a profound and destabilizing shock, leaving patients struggling with initial reactions of disbelief and denial. Thoughts such as, "This simply cannot be accurate; I only presented with symptoms of indigestion," or "This is not happening to me," are common and understandable responses. In these challenging moments, a confirmatory evaluation by a competent and empathetic physician can prove invaluable. When the diagnosis is corroborated by a second independent assessment, it facilitates the patient's confrontation with and eventual acceptance of the unwelcome reality, thereby easing the transition to the subsequent phases of treatment.

A comparable scenario often arises with patients undergoing coronary angiography for the evaluation of cardiac symptoms. The detection of stenotic (narrowed) coronary arteries constitutes unwelcome news; however, if all three major coronary arteries are found to be significantly affected, and the attending cardiologist recommends coronary artery bypass graft surgery rather than percutaneous coronary intervention (angioplasty), the patient will typically seek a second opinion from another cardiac surgeon before consenting to the major surgical procedure.

"Doctor hopping" or "medical shopping," on the other hand, bears a closer resemblance to the process of procuring produce at a market—moving from vendor to vendor, inquiring about the price of cauliflower, scrutinizing its size and quality, and sometimes engaging in negotiation before making a purchase. Some individuals, driven by a habitual desire to secure the most economical option, may inquire about the cost of an endoscopic procedure at five different medical centers before selecting one. At other times, it is not solely the price but also the perceived prestige or popularity of the physician or the established reputation of the clinic that influences their decision-making.

I recall an instance involving a nouveau riche businessman's wife in her forties who presented with her 12-year-old daughter, who had been experiencing persistent abdominal pain for a month. The child, however, appeared perfectly comfortable, smiling and relaxed as she sat across from me. While reviewing the child's medical history and the numerous ultrasound and CT scans she had undergone, the mother proudly disclosed that she had consulted with 18 of the city's leading pediatricians, surgeons, and gastroenterologists prior to seeking my opinion.

During our conversation, I ascertained that the reported pain typically manifested in the mornings before school but invariably subsided once the child was permitted to remain at home, enabling her to subsequently accompany her mother on shopping excursions to the mall. By the conclusion of the consultation, I could discern a clear sense of disappointment etched on the mother's face as she departed with her daughter, presumably to pursue their 20th medical consultation.

"Profiling Patients"

I wonder how many people I've looked at all my life and never seen.
- John Steinbeck

My professional life as a physician exposes me to an extraordinarily broad spectrum of emotional experiences on a daily basis: ranging from profound gratitude and elation at one extreme, to deep frustration and sorrow at the other, and, with increasing frequency, to the disquieting sensation of being blamed and accused, a feeling I find hurting and difficult to overcome.

Consider the following patient archetypes, each of which elicits distinct emotional responses within me:

Type 1:

I recall a young woman who accompanied her elderly mother to my clinic, having traveled from a distant part of the city. My initial inquiry focused on the reason for their extensive journey, given the availability of reputable medical facilities closer to their residence. Her simple yet poignant response was, "I brought my father to you the previous year, and you successfully treated his bile duct obstruction. We place our trust solely in you." This patient profile represents the most gratifying category: individuals who are genuinely satisfied, demonstrably grateful, and exude warmth, inspiring us to invest our utmost efforts in their care.

Type 2:

Experiences of sadness and frustration are unfortunately not uncommon within our profession. I remember a young man who brought his elderly and infirm mother to me, as she was suffering from an episode of severe acute pancreatitis. Despite three weeks of intensive care in an ICU, mechanical ventilation, and significant financial expenditure, she ultimately succumbed to her illness despite our best efforts. The family was understandably devastated by their loss. That evening, I recall canceling a social engagement, as I felt a deep sense of sorrow and empathy for the bereaved family.

Type 3:

A 65-year-old businessman presented to my clinic with liver cirrhosis secondary to years of excessive alcohol consumption. He had previously been hospitalized to manage ascites (fluid accumulation in the abdomen) and pleural effusions (fluid around the lungs), from which we had successfully facilitated his recovery. Despite our emphatic recommendations to abstain from alcohol, he resumed consumption shortly after discharge from hospital. Our attempts to assist him in achieving sobriety proved unsuccessful. I provided both verbal and written warnings regarding the health consequences, prescribed medications to mitigate alcohol cravings, arranged counseling sessions with addiction specialists, while his family attempted to exert emotional influence. This confluence of factors created a fertile ground for the "blame game." The family members held us accountable for our perceived inability to prevent his relapse, while I felt that the family was not investing sufficient time and effort in supporting his recovery. A sense of frustration ensued, and I could not help but anticipate potential negative repercussions.

Type 4:

A media executive entered my office, accompanied by a legal professional. Without uttering a word, he activated the recording function on his mobile phone and presented me with a thick file containing numerous investigative reports—most of which revealed no significant abnormalities. I immediately sensed his underlying anger, suspicion, and a palpable sense of depression. As our consultation progressed, I learned that his family was experiencing significant internal conflict and that his son, a high school dropout, was undergoing therapy for addiction and depression. His demeanor was discourteous and accusatory. He spoke disparagingly about the ten physicians he had consulted prior to seeking my opinion. It was evident that I was likely to be added to his growing list of "bad doctors". I chose to maintain a strictly professional demeanor, responding to his inquiries with precise technical details. However, I refrained from expressing any personal empathy for his difficult circumstances or offering well-intentioned advice regarding how he might improve his personal life and find greater happiness. I recognized that such advice could be easily misconstrued or misinterpreted. Ultimately, I suggested that he consult with another senior physician if my recommended treatment approach did not yield the desired results—a likely outcome, in my assessment.

***

The patient-physician relationship transcends the transactional nature of a typical consumer-seller interaction, such as purchasing a commonplace item like a toothbrush. It represents a profoundly personal and human connection, where the patient's attitude, disposition, and engagement play an equally vital role in fostering a therapeutic alliance and achieving positive health outcomes.

Doctors: The New Scapegoats

" The scapegoat is the child that can never do anything right. No matter what he does. It is never good enough"

Within the multifaceted roles we assume as physicians—encompassing healer, comforter, mentor, and educator—one frequently overlooked yet profoundly significant function is that of a scapegoat, serving as a psychological punching bag for displaced emotions.

Consider the case of 45-year-old Rahul (a pseudonym employed to protect privacy), who experienced a sudden collapse at his residence after a significant episode of hematemesis, vomiting two liters of blood. He was immediately transported to our hospital; however, despite our concerted efforts, he tragically succumbed to his condition within two hours of arrival. His family subsequently directed their grief and anger towards our medical team and the institution, alleging negligence and administrative failings.

Rahul's demise was a consequence of complications arising from decompensated liver cirrhosis, a condition that had progressively developed over two decades of chronic alcohol abuse. It must have been an intensely painful and frustrating ordeal for his parents to witness their son's gradual decline, despite their repeated attempts to steer him away from detrimental influences, including association with delinquent peers and the adoption of destructive habits. Yet, they did not assign culpability to themselves, their son, or his social associates for his self-destructive behavior.

Instead, they externalized their grief and placed the onus of responsibility upon us, holding a 10 minutes delay in starting blood transfusion as the cause of death. I came to understand that by selecting an external object for their blame, the family unconsciously established a mechanism to maintain emotional cohesion and solidarity during their profound grief and bereavement.

Scapegoating, therefore, is the perpetrator's defence mechanism against unacceptable emotions such as shame and guilt.

The phenomenon of scapegoating, or "blame transfer," is a common occurrence in the patient-physician dynamic, often enacted by patients without conscious awareness. When a chronic smoker develops bronchogenic carcinoma (lung cancer), culpability is typically assigned to the tobacco industry. If the malignancy is diagnosed at an advanced stage, the onus of responsibility shifts to the initial physician who may have overlooked the persistent cough and failed to recommend a bronchoscopy. And if the patient ultimately succumbs to the disease, the oncology specialist and the hospital are held accountable for not achieving a curative outcome. Within this cycle of blame, everyone is deemed at fault—with the notable exception of the smoker himself, his family, or those who were enablers of the detrimental behavior.

In another illustrative case, a 29-year-old man, exhibiting considerable frustration and anger, consulted me regarding chronic constipation. He recounted having consulted five different physicians over the preceding year, each of whom had prescribed mild, fiber-based laxatives under various brand names. While these interventions had provided symptomatic relief, he now reproached the physicians for having made him "dependent" on psyllium husk (Isabgol).

Through careful questioning, I ascertained that he had relinquished a stable employment position two years prior to pursue his ambition of becoming an officer in the Indian Administrative Service. When I inquired about a contingency plan in the event that his aspirations were not realized, he became visibly distressed and emotional. Through tears, he confided that if he failed to achieve his career goals, he intended to hold the physicians and the laxatives responsible for his perceived failure.

Patients often operate under the assumption that they are entitled to "receive" health and even life itself from us, without acknowledging the potential contributions of their own behaviors and circumstances to their health status. When desired outcomes are not achieved, there is a psychological need to externalize their shortcomings or guilt and assign blame to an external entity—to identify a scapegoat. And who is most readily available to fulfill this role? We physicians, of course.

As a physician, it is crucial to recognize this unique tendency among deeply distressed patients and their families to paradoxically direct blame toward us, rather than expressing gratitude for our efforts. While such reactions can be disheartening, it is important to remind ourselves that they frequently originate from the individual's experience of pain, fear, and a sense of helplessness. By cultivating an understanding of this particular psychological need, one can respond with greater kindness, empathy, and equanimity, maintaining professional composure and compassion in the face of these challenging interactions.

Be kind to your patients, inspite of them pointing fingers at you. Understand that they are coming from a position of deep pain and helplessness at that moment.

Should Doctors Lie for their Patients?

A Truth can walk naked, but a lie always needs to be dressed.

-Khalil Gibran

"It was not the truth they wanted, but an illusion they could bear to live with"

Anais Nin

I frequently find myself in ethically challenging situations with patients when they pose the timeless question, "Is telling a lie always morally reprehensible?" The above two quotations point to the need for a good doctor to choose the person, context and occasion with discretion.

As an individual who firmly believes in the public's role as the moral compass of society, I seek your opinion. I will present some of the dilemmas I have encountered, hoping to gain valuable insights from your perspectives.

Case 1:

My initial encounter with this ethical quandary occurred 35 years ago when a young nurse, approximately 30 years of age, consulted me regarding frequent episodes of watery stools since the morning. After promptly writing a prescription for presumed infective diarrhea and advising her to take two days of medical leave, she expressed her gratitude and began to depart.

She then paused and explained that she required the leave to travel to her hometown, located 200 kilometers away, to retrieve her young child from her parents' care, explaining that no one else was available to undertake this task.

"But what about your loose stools?" I inquired, taken aback.

"Actually, I don't have any loose stools. I simply needed the leave, as I have exhausted all of my other leave options!" she admitted candidly.

I experienced a mixture of shock and unease. I instinctively retrieved the prescription from her hand and began to invalidate it.

"Doctor, please advise me on what other course of action I could have taken? Are you not effectively penalizing me for being honest?" she attempted to justify her actions.

This presented a significant ethical dilemma. Had she maintained her initial assertion of having diarrhea, I would have readily granted her the requested leave. However, her subsequent honesty had disturbed my moral conscience.

I carefully considered the potential ramifications of both courses of action. If I granted her the leave, I would be implicitly condoning a deception. Conversely, if I refused her request, I would be discouraging her honesty and potentially incentivizing future dishonesty.

What would be the ethically justifiable course of action? Should I acquiesce to a minor deception? Or should I uphold strict adherence to truthfulness?

What would you do in this situation?

Case 2:

A 40-year-old clerical worker was admitted to the hospital due to an episode of severe acute pancreatitis. Upon admission, he disclosed to the on-duty physician that he had consumed alcohol at a social gathering the previous day. However, after he subsequently lapsed into a comatose state, his family members vehemently denied any knowledge of his alcohol consumption. His condition progressively deteriorated, necessitating intensive care unit admission for 15 days, incurring substantial medical expenses totaling Rs 10 lakh. Despite all medical interventions and financial resources expended, he ultimately passed away.

His distraught, semi-literate wife and their three school-aged children were left in a precarious financial situation. They had incurred significant debt, sold their ancestral land in their village, and now faced the imminent threat of destitution.

In the midst of their profound distress and vulnerability, they implored me to omit any mention of alcohol consumption from the initial medical report, as they were convinced that such a disclosure would almost certainly result in the insurance company rejecting their medical claim.

What should I do in this ethically complex situation? Should I acquiesce to their request and potentially falsify medical documentation? Or should I adhere strictly to factual reporting, despite the potential for severe financial hardship for the bereaved family?

What would you do?

***

Many readers might consider these ethical dilemmas to be relatively minor and may invoke the example of the virtuous Yudhisthira from the Mahabharata, whose unwavering adherence to truth throughout his life ultimately led to his ascension to heaven. However, we physicians are mere mortals, and unlike the mythical Yudhisthira, we often find ourselves in situations where strict adherence to absolute truth presents significant challenges and complex ramifications.

Legends of Healthcare

Eternal Icons of Nursing

In the absence of purpose, life becomes an endless journey to nowhere.
-Seneca

It is difficult to envision healthcare institutions functioning without nurses; however, their crucial contributions to patient care often remain underappreciated. Let us briefly delve into the historical context of this essential profession and trace its evolution.

The narrative commences with Florence Nightingale, an Englishwoman born on May 12, 1820, in Florence, Italy, where her parents were celebrating their honeymoon. Upon their return to England, she pursued studies in literature, history, philosophy, and mathematics, eventually developing expertise in statistical analysis. Despite her status as a refined English lady, she demonstrated no interest in the numerous marriage proposals she received from the age of 17.

She derived profound solace from her religious convictions as a member of the Protestant Christian faith and felt a deep, intrinsic calling to serve and provide care for those afflicted by suffering. In 1850, she underwent formal nursing training in Germany and subsequently began providing fundamental nursing care in hospitals throughout England and continental Europe.

Her opportunity to provide large-scale patient care arose during the Crimean War, a conflict between Russia and the Ottoman Empire. British and Allied forces joined with the Ottomans in a fierce struggle on the

Crimean Peninsula. While many soldiers perished in combat, an even greater number suffered and died in overcrowded and unsanitary military hospitals due to the absence of adequate medical care. Responding to this dire humanitarian crisis, Florence Nightingale organized and led a contingent of British nurses, embarking on a voyage in October 1854 and arriving at the Scutari Barrack Hospital on November 5 of the same year.

The subsequent events are well-documented: a small team of 38 dedicated young British nurses began tending to wounded British soldiers, many of whom were succumbing to infectious diseases rather than direct combat injuries. Their tireless efforts contributed to the recovery and survival of countless soldiers. Florence Nightingale earned the enduring moniker "The Lady with the Lamp" as she diligently patrolled the hospital wards, carrying a lamp, amidst the pervasive stench of gangrene and the suffering of dying soldiers, attending to all those she could assist.

She authored over 200 books and pamphlets, emphasizing the crucial role of a clean and sanitary environment and compassionate care in the healing process. She championed the advancement of nursing education and standardized training protocols, as well as the implementation of efficient hospital planning and organizational structures. Universally recognized as the "Pioneer of Modern Nursing," Florence Nightingale left an enduring legacy, including the establishment of the British Red Cross in 1870 and the creation of the first dedicated Department of Nursing at St. Thomas' Hospital in London, an institution established in her honor.

Her astute observations, substantiated by meticulous statistical data, remain remarkably relevant in contemporary healthcare settings. She underscored the importance of maintaining a clean hospital environment, ensuring proper ventilation, providing hygienic bedding, maintaining sanitary kitchen facilities, and offering nutritious meals. She also prioritized the emotional well-being of patients by facilitating communication between wounded soldiers and their loved ones through letter writing and establishing reading rooms to bolster their morale. Alongside these practical contributions, she established the foundational principles for the discipline and methodologies of modern nursing practice.

What resonates most profoundly with me is her holistic approach, seamlessly integrating scientific nursing interventions with profound empathy and compassion.

Her later years were marked by hardship; she was largely confined to her bed for three decades until her death in 1910, likely due to a chronic infection contracted during her service to wounded soldiers.

However, even today, she remains the singular guiding light of modern nursing worldwide, with healthcare professionals of all disciplines—nurses, physicians, and hospital administrators—drawing inspiration from her exceptional contributions, selfless service, unwavering dedication, remarkable foresight, and enduring impact on global healthcare.

***

While Florence Nightingale justly occupies a preeminent position as a pioneering figure in nursing history, it is essential to acknowledge the numerous other individuals who made substantial contributions to the profession. Recognizing and commemorating their achievements serves to inspire and motivate successive generations of nurses.

Figures such as Clara Barton, who served as a nurse during the American Civil War and subsequently founded the American Red Cross, and Dorothea Dix, an educator and social reformer who dedicated her life to advocating for and improving the welfare of individuals with mental illness, have also left an indelible mark on healthcare. Margaret Sanger, renowned for her compassionate work in maternal health and family planning, is another noteworthy example, among a multitude of others.

In the Indian context, Bai Kashibai Ganpat holds a significant place in nursing history as the first Indian woman to formally enter the profession. In 1891, she graduated from JJ Hospital in Mumbai, at a time when societal attitudes in India closely mirrored those of Victorian England, the era in which Florence Nightingale discerned her calling to dedicate herself to nursing and the care of the sick. Bai Kashibai Ganpat's unwavering dedication, pioneering spirit, and commitment to service effectively opened pathways for numerous women in India to pursue careers in nursing, thereby playing a pivotal role in elevating the profession to its present standing.

Ms. Shanti Teresa Lakra stands as another remarkable Indian nursing professional who made substantial contributions to the field of nursing in India. Often recognized as the "Florence Nightingale of India," she dedicated herself to providing care for the Onge tribe in the Andaman and Nicobar Islands in the aftermath of the devastating 2004 Indian Ocean tsunami. Her extraordinary service and unwavering commitment to the affected communities garnered widespread recognition, culminating in her being awarded the Padma Shri, one of India's highest civilian honors, in 2011, for her exceptional dedication and selfless contributions to healthcare.

***

In contemporary healthcare, the professional landscape for nurses has undergone a significant transformation, presenting novel challenges and responsibilities that diverge considerably from those encountered in previous generations.

It is not uncommon to encounter clinical scenarios in which a critically ill patient, initially deemed to have a poor prognosis, is successfully operated upon by a team of highly specialized surgeons and subsequently resuscitated and stabilized by intensivists within the intensive care unit. After a period of weeks in the hospital, during which hope for recovery is restored, the patient may unexpectedly succumb to complications, such as an adverse drug reaction following an incorrectly administered injection or a healthcare-associated infection originating from an indwelling catheter—events that can often be attributed to a lapse in nursing care. In such tragic circumstances, the patient's family members experience a profound sense of betrayal and intense anger, emotions that rapidly supplant the preceding weeks of gratitude and appreciation for the seemingly heroic medical interventions.

A further exacerbating factor within busy and understaffed hospital settings is the frequent lack of both time and specialized training afforded to nurses to provide adequate emotional support and bereavement counseling to grieving relatives during these critical junctures. Consequently, these bereaved family members often depart the hospital with enduringly negative recollections and a sense of profound dissatisfaction with the care provided.

Frankly, excessive demands are often placed upon nurses, while insufficient attention is given to their own well-being and professional support. Many hospitals operate with critically low nursing staff levels, which inevitably leads to the overworking and burnout of the remaining nursing personnel.

Too much is expected out of understaffed, overworked and uncared for nurses!

Consider the typical workload of nurses: a standard evening or night shift often consists of just two nurses tasked with caring for 30, and in some instances, as many as 60, acutely ill patients over a period of six to eight hours. While this may initially seem manageable, a closer examination of their responsibilities reveals a significantly more demanding reality. During this shift, they are typically expected to:

- Receive a handover of medication stock and patient information from the preceding shift (approximately 30 minutes).
- Monitor each patient's vital signs (pulse rate, blood pressure, respiration, and temperature) every four to six hours (approximately 10 minutes per patient x 30 patients = 300 minutes, or five hours).
- Administer medications (which are highly individualized based on patient needs) to 30 patients every two to six hours (approximately 90 minutes).
- Administer injections to approximately 20 patients.
- Collect blood samples for laboratory testing from approximately 10 patients.
- Initiate intravenous fluid infusions or change existing IV fluid bags for approximately 15 patients.
- Transport patients for various procedures, such as surgery, endoscopy, or radiology (approximately 10 patients).

- Assist physicians with minor bedside procedures, such as ascitic or pleural fluid aspiration (approximately 10 patients).
- Oversee patient dietary intake.
- Complete discharge paperwork and provide discharge instructions to departing patients.

And this list is not exhaustive.

In addition to these routine tasks, nurses must also be prepared to respond to acute patient deteriorations, assisting with resuscitation efforts (which can take approximately 30 minutes per incident) and responding to frequent emergency calls, given that a substantial proportion (often around 50%) of the patient population within the ward consists of critically ill individuals.

A careful analysis of their actual workload during a typical shift reveals the remarkable feat they accomplish simply to meet basic patient needs. This raises a critical question: where, within this demanding schedule, is there time for the essential components of compassionate nursing care—providing emotional support and establishing rapport with patients and their families, attending to personal hygiene needs such as bathing and skin care, and performing all the other acts of kindness and attentiveness that constitute truly excellent nursing?

It is fundamentally unfair to expect nurses to consistently perform at a superhuman level throughout their careers. While the complexity and intensity of medical care have increased exponentially over the past five decades, the nurse-to-patient ratio has remained largely stagnant. Strengthening this critical pillar of the healthcare system through increased staffing and support is absolutely essential if we are to achieve meaningful improvements in the quality of hospital care.

Its time to create a nurturing ambiance for our nurses to make way for compassion to seep back into healthcare.

The nursing profession offers a unique and invaluable opportunity to serve and care for individuals experiencing suffering, placing nurses in a prime position to embody the very qualities of empathy and compassion that are increasingly absent within contemporary healthcare and society at large. Consequently, nurses require focused attention, robust support systems, consistent nurturing, genuine empowerment, and effective leadership if the healthcare sector is to progress and achieve higher standards of patient care. While nursing training institutions play a crucial role in foundational education, practical learning, as is widely acknowledged within the healthcare field, truly commences after graduation—at the patient's bedside, through direct clinical experience.

Mother Teresa: Personification of Empathy

I call him religious who understands the suffering of others.
-Mahatma Gandhi

The centenary of Mother Teresa's birth served as a global commemoration of her enduring legacy as an icon of selfless care and unwavering compassion for the sick and impoverished. Her life and work provide an unparalleled source of inspiration for medical professionals to integrate empathy into their daily practice. While prominent images of Mother Teresa frequently grace the walls of hospitals, it is a poignant paradox that the very essence of her profound humanity often appears to be absent among the personnel within those institutions.

In a not-so-distant past, physicians and nurses had limited therapeutic interventions at their disposal, their primary offerings to patients consisted of personal attention, comfort, genuine compassion, and sincere concern for their afflictions. Medical practitioners were held in high regard and earned considerable respect for whatever palliative care they could provide for conditions then deemed incurable.

What was the driving force behind Mother Teresa's extraordinary dedication? Her establishment for the sick and destitute, Nirmal Hriday (meaning "Pure Heart"), frequently operated at capacity and lacked sophisticated medical infrastructure. Indeed, she faced criticism during her lifetime for managing a hospice with limited resources. Despite these material constraints, individuals in need sought refuge there, receiving not advanced medical procedures, but rather profound expressions of love and devoted care, allowing them to spend their final days with dignity and a sense of peace. Their passing was often marked by a serene sense of acceptance. Remarkably, their families did not resort to verbal aggression towards the staff or initiate legal proceedings. The distinguishing characteristic of Nirmal Hriday was not the sophistication of its medical technology or the availability of advanced treatments, but rather the pervasive atmosphere of love, empathy, and compassion that pervaded every interaction, transforming a simple, unassuming setting into a sanctuary of tranquility and solace.

I vividly recall listening to her Nobel Peace Prize acceptance address in 1979, in which her discourse centered almost exclusively on the transformative power of love. Nirmal Hriday was characterized as "a place of hope, a house built on courage and faith, a home where love reigns, a home filled with love." How deeply I yearn for our contemporary hospitals to be able to make such a statement about themselves. Her counsel to her staff was both simple and deeply resonant: "Let no one who comes to you ever leave without feeling happier and better."

Could we not, as physicians and members of the broader healthcare community, endeavor to incorporate this principle into our professional ethos?

Dr. Binyak Sen: Rebel or Saviour?

Love and compassion are necessities, not luxuries. Without them, humanity cannot survive.

- Dalai Lama

For those unfamiliar with his background, Dr. Binayak Sen is not a conventional, politically motivated physician. He is a specialist in Pediatrics and Public Health, with teaching experience at Jawaharlal Nehru University in Delhi. His formative experiences likely began during his time at the esteemed Christian Medical College (CMC), Vellore, one of the few institutions that continues to emphasize humanistic values and a spirit of social service among its students. His research on "Marasmus and Malnutrition in Children" led to a deeper engagement with the interconnected issues of hunger, poverty, malnutrition, and the devastating impact on the lives of impoverished children.

Dr. Sen, who dedicated his life to serving the impoverished and marginalized tribal communities of Chhattisgarh, soon recognized that poverty and starvation were the fundamental causes of malnutrition among children in rural India. He understood that expensive protein and vitamin supplements could not provide a sustainable solution for impoverished rural India ("Bharat"), a world far removed from the affluent, globally recognized, and commercially prosperous sections. The Christian ethos instilled during his training at CMC likely cultivated a deep sense of altruism in this committed young physician, prompting a profound moral conflict as he witnessed children in nearby slums suffering from starvation, moaning in pain, and crying for sustenance.

What would have constituted the ethically sound course of action for him? To disregard the pervasive misery, establish a lucrative private practice in a fashionable urban setting, prescribe vitamin supplements for well-nourished children from affluent families, engage in leisurely pursuits such as snooker, and participate in social gatherings over alcoholic beverages, as many within the profession choose to do?

We physicians experience our own unique blend of joys, challenges, and frustrations. It is difficult to articulate the profound sense of fulfillment we derive when a critically ill child triumphs over adversity and offers a heartfelt expression of gratitude through a smile before returning home. Conversely, it is equally frustrating to witness the loss of a life when a potentially curative intervention is just beyond reach due to scarcity of resources, food, essential medications, or even basic supportive care.

How does one respond to the pleading gaze of a child afflicted with tuberculosis, further debilitated by the combined burdens of malnutrition and poverty? How does one convey to tribal laborers, who lack the financial means for treatment, that allowing their child to die might represent a form of mercy for both the child and their remaining family members? And what if the financial resources required to save the child represented a mere fraction of the funds expended by the child's employer on extravagant social events? In such a context, would a desperate act of bending or breaking a rule to save the child's life constitute a heinous transgression?

In 2004, Binayak Sen received the Paul Harrison Award from the Christian Medical College, Vellore, in recognition of his exceptional contributions to society, "for carrying his dedication to service to the very frontline of battle and for redefining the possible role of the doctor in a broken and unjust society."

If this constitutes a crime, should physicians not feel a sense of pride in committing it repeatedly?

Celebrating Doctors' Day: Honouring Dr. Bidhan Chandra Roy

No act of kindness, no matter how small, is ever wasted.

-Aesop

July 1st marks Doctors' Day in India—a day dedicated to celebrating, honoring, and expressing appreciation for the unwavering dedication and tireless efforts of physicians across the nation.

The concept appears to have originated in the state of Georgia, USA, where appreciative patients, their families, and the wider community utilized the occasion to express their gratitude to physicians by sending cards to them and their spouses (acknowledging the significant sacrifices made by doctors' families) or even by placing floral tributes on the graves of these benefactors.

Many countries now observe their own designated Doctors' Day. However, the motivations and methods of celebration have evolved considerably—shifting from expressions of genuine gratitude and heartfelt emotion from citizens to more formalized forms of awards and recognition conferred by the healthcare industry, media organizations, or government bodies.

The specific date chosen for Doctors' Day in India commemorates the birth anniversary of one of the country's most distinguished physicians, Dr. Bidhan Chandra Roy.

The life story of Dr.Bidhan Chandra Roy, also known as B.C. Roy, after whom the prestigious national awards for exceptional achievements in medicine are named, serves as a powerful source of inspiration. He was born on this day in 1882 in Patna, where he received his early education. He subsequently pursued his medical training in Calcutta (now Kolkata) and later traveled to England for advanced studies.

Remarkably, his application for admission to St. Bartholomew's Hospital (St Bart's) in London was reportedly rejected by the dean on 30 separate occasions before finally being accepted, demonstrating his extraordinary perseverance and unwavering determination. He then attained both his Membership of the Royal College of Physicians (MRCP) and Fellowship of the Royal College of Surgeons (FRCS) qualifications in just over two years before returning to India.

Early in his professional career, he served in the provincial medical service while also maintaining a private practice, charging a consultation fee of Rs 8. He later served as a faculty member at Calcutta Medical College for several years.

He entered the political arena in 1925 and steadily progressed to become the Chief Minister of West Bengal. During his long tenure in this role, numerous hospitals and clinics were established in Kolkata, which continue to form the cornerstone of the state's public health infrastructure.

Dr. Roy was a visionary leader; he endeavored to decentralize development within West Bengal, which had previously been concentrated primarily in Calcutta, and spearheaded the development of several new towns, including Durgapur, Kalyani, and Bidhan Nagar.

He remained unmarried, dedicating his personal resources to the welfare of the state, and passed away at the age of 80 on his birth date, July 1st. He was posthumously awarded the Bharat Ratna, India's highest civilian honor, in 1961.

The observance of a commemorative day such as Doctors' Day is a worthwhile endeavor. Although physicians in India have at times been portrayed negatively in the media, receiving numerous phone calls, cards, and messages of appreciation from grateful patients and their families on this particular day is genuinely heartwarming and reinforces our conviction that choosing this profession was indeed a fulfilling and meaningful decision.

Epilogue

Writing this book has been a deeply personal journey. In sharing these stories, I've revisited moments of profound joy, heartbreaking loss, and everything in between. I've been reminded of the immense privilege it is to walk alongside people during some of the most vulnerable moments of their lives. And I've learned, time and time again, that caring is not a one-way street. The moments I've spent caring for others have also profoundly provided care to my soul, soothed my conscience and shaped me into the doctor, and the loved person, I am today. My hope is that these reflections will stay with you long after you've closed this book, and that they will inspire you to embrace the transformative power of caring in your own life.

And a doctor, perhaps more than any other in society, needs to remind himself of Langland's quote, every day he tends to a patient"

" We should be low and love like and lean each man to other. And patient as pilgrim for pilgrims are we all."

-`William Langland

References

References for Facilitating Graceful Death and Caregiving:

- *End of Life Care: Living Will - Advanced medical directive, Information booklet-Indian medical Association, Goa*
- *Advance Medical Directive (living will) and health care power-of-attorney authorisation*
- *Advance Medical Directive Toolkit*
- *End-of-life Care Toolkit- VIDHI Centre for Legal Policy*
- *Rx for Resilience by Dr Saroj Dubey*
- *Curbside consultation and other anecdotes by Dr Anil C Anand*
- *UN-USUAL People- A caregiver's manual by Aldred L Anduze*
- *The Joyful Caregiver- 8 steps to prevent caregiver burnout by Josephine Grace*
- *The Home Stretch: A Family Caregiver's Handbook by Sanjay Dattatri*
- *Health Adda by Dr Gourdas Choudhuri*

Other books by the author (Available on Amazon/ Flipkart)

- *Health Adda (Notion Press)*
- *Ten Steps to Good Health (Bloomsbury)*

Other technical books by the Author

- *Gastroenterology and Hepatology- Bench to Bedside (Springer)*
- *Non-Alcoholic Fatty Liver- Current concepts and Emerging Therapies (Converse)*
- *Atlas of Gastrointestinal Endoscopy* (*Medicca Press*)
- *Non-Alcoholic Fatty Liver disease: A Clinical Spectrum* (*Elsevier*)
- *Gastroesophageal Reflux Disease (Knowledge Bridge)*
- *Alcoholic Liver disease* (*Kontent Workx*)
- *Hepatitis* (*Elsevier*)

